P9-CKU-702

OVERCOMING THE MYTHS OF AGING

Lose Weight, Look Great and Live a Happier, Healthier Life

By
Roe Gallo, Ph.D.
and
Stephen Zocchi

Overcoming the Myths of Aging

Copyright 2007, Roe Gallo and Stephen Zocchi

Publishing by
Roe Gallo Publishing
P.O. Box 78096 San Francisco, CA 94107
www.roegallo.com

Photography
Lisa Leigh Photography
www.lisaleigh.com
469 Miller Avenue
Mill Valley, CA 94941
415-389-0609

Cover Design
MindSWEEP, Inc.
www.mindsweep.ca
475 Acadie Avenue
Acadie, Dieppe, NB, E1A 1H7
t. 506-855-4695 x222 - f. 506-855-2879 - c. 506-866-5468

Book Design
Nick Nyffeler - Graphic Designer
nicknyffeler@hotmail.com

Printed in the United States of America.

Printed on recycled paper with soy-based ink by
Alonzo Printing
3266 Investment Blvd. Hayward, CA 94545
510-293-0522
www.alonzoprinting.com

ISBN 10: 0-9642253-1-X
ISBN 13: 978-0-9642253-1-2

Disclaimer

Overcoming the Myths of Aging and the OTM plan are based on the concepts of physiology and exercise physiology and complement the natural functions of how the body works. Roe Gallo and Stephen Zocchi are not medical doctors nor do they claim to be. They do not practice medicine.

Remember, when embarking on any new health and fitness program it is sometimes wise to get some coaching from your personal health and/or fitness professionals.

Also, there are many great books written by professionals in the health and fitness field that can also provide additional insights that complement the ideas in this book, some great ones are listed in the bibliography.

It ain't what you don't know that gets you into trouble.

mark twain

It's what you know for sure that just ain't so.

TABLE OF CONTENTS

Stephen:

It's normal to expect that we'll gain some weight, do a bit less physical activity, or see our health erode. We are growing older after all. Why should we believe these signs of aging are myths?

Roe:

But is this "normal life" the life you want? Look around you. Everywhere you look you see more people who are rapidly aging, with more degenerative diseases, and much too much fat. Don't you want something better?

Now that I'm over 50 years old, I know my body is still doing its job—staying healthy and full of energy. Yet I see people my age and even younger suffering with poor health, lack of energy, and a lack of excitement and joy for life. Most of them blame it on aging, but it isn't aging. It's really about their lifestyle choices.

Stephen:

Well, the conventional wisdom doesn't support these ideas about aging being myths. It's not how we were raised, or what we were taught.

Roe:

Let's stop for a minute, and suspend the conditioning we've received over the years. What does common sense tell us when we see our friends, family, and society in general falling apart? The majority of the population is overweight and a large percentage is obese. This includes children and young adults.

The statistics are frightening:

According to the Center for Disease Control, between 1992 and 2001, doctor's visits for treatment of diabetes rose 63%.

The American Heart Association recently released these 2002 stats showing disease in baby boomers (those born between 1946 and 1963):

Over 36% have cardiovascular disease.

Over 31% have high blood pressure.

56% women and 60% men have high blood cholesterol.

65% women and 75% men are overweight.

37% women and 31% men are obese.

The rate of obesity has dramatically increased. For adults aged 20 years and older in 1960, the obesity rate was 10.7% and it had risen to 28% by 2002.

For the baby boomers, it increased from 15.7% to 34%. We are literally accelerating aging ourselves through bad diet, inactivity, and poor attitude.

Stephen:
It doesn't present too optimistic a picture, does it? We've worked hard for what we have achieved in life, and we are looking forward to living the wonderful life we deserve.

I guess I don't really feel old, so why should aging itself be an issue? What bothers me more are all the expected changes that are an accepted part of aging. I want more than that from the rest of my life.

Roe:
You should! These expectations you don't like are the myths of aging, and they are all around us. Most of us buy into the idea that as we get older, we will get fatter, sicker, and flabbier; we'll lose sex drive and sex appeal; and that it's really too late for us to make any big changes. Believing in these myths makes it difficult, if not impossible, to take our lives in the direction we want to go.

Stephen:
For that reason, your ideas about health and nutrition are appealing, because they touch upon the very issues I am seeing and feeling about aging, but they contradict conventional wisdom.

Roe:

So, are we better off following conventional wisdom with our normal diets and normal attitudes? No, we are getting sicker and fatter. But we don't have to. We need to learn to disbelieve the conventional wisdom. More and more, the healthcare community is preaching diet and lifestyle changes, but why aren't we listening? We have the right information, but the biggest obstacle to doing it is believing it.

Stephen:

But when I read your last book, Perfect Body, I felt that your approach was so rigidly structured, so different, that it would be difficult—no, probably impossible—for me to follow.

Roe:

I was told many times that the original Perfect Body food plan was much too difficult to follow, mostly by people who were not in an apparent life-and-death situation.

Stephen:

That's most of us. I am looking for something that will keep me healthy and fit, yet not make me feel deprived or set me up for failure. I want to lose weight, look great, and have a happier and healthier life for the rest of my life, but I want to do it my way and on my terms.

Roe:

Yes, but are you willing to disbelieve the myths of aging?

Stephen:

Based upon what I learned in Perfect Body, I could be ready, but is there a way to get most of the benefits of your approach with more flexibility? I think that would help more people like me defeat the myths of aging.

Roe:

Maybe you could help me. You are asking the questions that most people ask. You could be the voice of reality. With your input, we can build a plan that is suited for a wider audience. A plan for everyday life that is based upon choice and not driven by mandate. A plan that can help everyone overcome these myths of aging.

Stephen:

A plan for overcoming the myths…how about calling it the OTM plan?

Roe:

Great! And, like Perfect Body, the OTM plan will focus on improving the entire body and mind. A program that will extend beyond just food and nutrition. But what do you think we need to tell people to help them dispel the myths for themselves?

Stephen:

When I read your story – what led you to develop the "Perfect Body" plan – that got me thinking. Start with that. Then I would help people see for themselves how the myths of aging are myths, and what they can do about it in a way that can fit their own unique life style.

OVERCOMING
My Myths

They stood over my bed, shaking their heads.

In that moment I knew my medical team was not sure. They were guessing. They didn't know what to do, and I knew I had to get out of there. For 25 years, I had entrusted my life to a group of people who I now saw were basically clueless—at least as it pertained to my situation. But what could I do? How could I escape the outcome they were leading me toward? I was in a wheelchair, my breathing wasn't strong enough to allow me to walk, I could not breathe at all without the drugs or could I?

I remembered my father's mother. She was kind and loving, but also strong and determined. She had a stroke and was paralyzed on her left side. Her doctor told her she would never walk again, but she didn't believe them. Instead, she would push herself out of bed, desperately trying to walk. She did this every day until she was able to walk again. I was very much like my grandmother—we even looked alike.

I had been in the hospital for a month. It seemed like years. I had a severe allergic reaction at a restaurant and had gone into anaphylactic shock. I was rushed to the nearest hospital, and in the emergency room I was injected with adrenaline. After the adrenaline took effect, I was given aminophylline, a new asthma drug. I've had a life long struggle with asthma. The next thing I remember was being slapped and yelled at. The group of doctors surrounding me was administering more adrenaline. My heart had stopped; my body had rejected the aminophylline.

After I was stable, I was transported to the pulmonary ward for further treatment. At the time of my admittance I could walk, but after less than two weeks in the ward I could barely push my own wheelchair. By the end of the third week, my pain was so great, and my breathing so shallow, I couldn't even wheel myself down the hall. I asked the doctors why I was getting worse, but they told me not to worry—that I would improve in time. But I was worried. I was confused and intuitively I knew that something was very wrong. I wondered if it might be my medication, so I asked the medical staff about my medication. I was told not to worry and they gave me no further information. I was becoming terrified from watching and feeling my body fall apart. So I decided I had to investigate on my own.

I asked a fellow patient to wheel me to the nurses' station and, when no one was looking, I examined my chart. The doctors were prescribing an oral dose of aminophylline, the same medication they gave me in the emergency room that had caused my heart to stop.

Did my medical team know? Did they not read my chart? Was I reading my chart wrong? I had been raised to trust medical professionals completely. How could this be happening? How could there be such an apparent contradiction? My medical team, after a lot of head shaking, admitted that they were aware that the drug was the same, but they considered it the best medication for me. They said the small, oral doses would not affect my body as had the larger, intravenous dose.

I felt myself on the path to a slow death versus a fast one! I could feel a growing sense of panic and loss of hope. I realized I needed to take control in order to save my own life.

I made a decision that I was going to get out of the hospital alive. Acting on my intuition and against my conditioning, I stopped taking all the medications. I began to palm the meds and pretend to take my doses. As soon as the nurse left, I would throw out the meds. I visualized the pain leaving my body. I took long showers and visualized my lungs clean. I drank large quantities of water to flush the drugs from my system. I ate only the fruits and vegetables that my friends brought to me. I never told anyone at the hospital what I was doing.

With each passing day, my medical team remarked on the

wonderful progress I was making. I said nothing but continued my regimen. Within one week I could walk well enough to sign myself out of the hospital. My doctors were upset. They tried to convince me to stay. They couldn't understand why I wanted to leave when I was finally improving. I was convinced that I was on to something, something that would help me. I knew the path I needed to take to save my life. I was still in pain, but I managed to get out of the hospital against the advice of my doctors and against the wishes of my family.

Even after this experience, I went to see a pulmonary specialist at the University of Pennsylvania. It was hard to break the patterns of a lifetime. He gave me a prescription for prednisone, a corticosteroid drug. Each time I took it, I initially experienced a day or two of relief. But by the third day, my pain would come back and breathing would again become difficult. My doctor's solution was to increase the dosage. I continued this treatment plan for three weeks. But I was in pain, still wheezing, and beginning to bloat. I looked up prednisone in the *Physician's Desk Reference (PDR)*. I discovered that it was classified as a "dependent" drug—the more I took, the more my body needed for survival. Eventually this drug too would kill me.

The next day I called my specialist to ask him about my findings. I could feel him shaking his head over the phone. Yes, he finally admitted, it was true; however, if I stopped the pills, I would die. I had faced this dilemma before. There had to be another way.

I recalled a course I'd recently completed in critical thinking. In this course, we had to examine media—films, books, news articles, etc., to find errors in logic. I did well in this class and now it seemed time to apply this learning to my life. I knew this meant that by taking charge of my life, I also would be taking charge of decisions concerning my death. I went to the local health-food stores (this was back in 1975, before Google) and looked at alternatives. Nothing made sense. Most of the books talked about plans that contradicted each other. I didn't have time to experiment. Instead, I read about the body's immune system and how it was designed to rid itself of toxins. I decided to take the chance on trusting my own body.

I threw out the pills!

All my childhood I was sick. I spent most of my younger years in bed or visiting the doctor. I suffered from severe, constant colds; headaches; and several bouts of pneumonia. I was allergic to dust, animals, pollen—almost everything. I couldn't live the lifestyle my friends took for granted. I couldn't run and play with the "normal" kids, because my chest would constrict with pain and I would wheeze and gasp for breath. I was a chronic asthmatic.

Doctors injected me with whatever the pharmaceutical companies were pushing that year. On days when I was well enough to go to school, I carried an inhaler and a well-stocked pillbox. I was a walking medicine cabinet. I endured chronic eczema, an irritating and embarrassing condition for which I was given medicated soaps, special lotions, artificial light applications, and numerous other treatments that never helped. That was how I grew up. That was the life I knew—my normal life.

After being hospitalized for anaphylactic shock, and contrary to all professional advice, I put my life in my own hands because I believed I could be healthy.

I did most of my research in the area of physiology, the study of how the body functions. When I studied the immune system, I was hopeful. I learned that toxicity was the key component for disease. I learned how the body is constantly trying to rid itself of waste, which is poisonous to the body. I decided that the only logical way to heal my body once and for all was to allow it to purge the toxins quickly before they finally killed me.

After 25 years of pain and suffering and coming close to death so many times, it only took my body two weeks to clean up the asthma. I can still remember the first deep breath I took without pain.

I learned so much from that experience.

I learned how to build a healthy immune system. I discovered that a strong immune system is extremely capable of keeping us healthy.

I learned about the power of the mind, the importance of a positive attitude and how to change negative, erroneous, and harmful beliefs into positive, accurate, and powerful ones.

I learned the power of decision. I decided that I was going to get out of the hospital alive and I was going to get healthy.

I learned there are three basic, yet extremely important, steps to changing our lives:

First, *get the correct information.*

Next, *believe in it.*

Finally, *live it.*

PERFECT
Body

In order to get control of my life back, I developed a plan for myself based around the research I did in physiology and good nutrition. I didn't have a choice. Well, actually I did, but that choice, to die from the medications, wasn't too appealing. The plan became my only alternative, and it worked.

Through my research and personal experience, I learned about toxicity and how that was the basic cause of my disease and much disease in general. I learned that by cleansing the body of toxins and keeping our internal fluids pure, we could get and stay healthy.

After some time I decided to share my plan because I knew there were others who were facing problems with their health and for whom the medical community had no good answers. I wrote a small book based on physiology and health called *Body Ecology*. When I was in graduate school, I expanded *Body Ecology* into *Perfect Body: The Raw Truth* and then revised it and changed the name slightly to *Perfect Body: Beyond the Illusion*.

My books focused on a plan based on fresh, raw, organic fruit and green leafy vegetables; distilled water, fresh squeezed citrus juice (orange, grapefruit) and not much else in the way of food. Of course, the plan wasn't just about food—it was about getting and staying healthy. Fitness, rest, sunshine, mental and emotional health, and a positive attitude toward life greatly affect our health too.

People who have searched for healthier diets and solutions to health problems found my Web site and ordered my book. *Perfect Body* was sent to England, France, Scotland, Greece, Germany,

Israel, Pakistan, Canada, Italy, China, Mexico, The Netherlands, Africa, Spain, Japan, Russia, and to other places that I'm probably not even aware of.

The *Perfect Body* plan was simple and effective. It worked if you did it, but doing it was the difficult part for most people. It hasn't surprised me that, over the past 20 plus years, the plan has succeeded in helping people live full and happy lives after recovering from heart disease, cancer, diabetes, asthma, and many other conditions. What did surprise me was how difficult it was for those who had no symptoms of disease to embrace the concepts in my plan. I couldn't understand their resistance—especially family and friends who knew me when I was sick. They watched as my life was transformed, yet they refused to consider a change. Or maybe they wanted to change, but it was just too difficult and without the pressing symptoms, they believed it was not really necessary.

Overcoming the Myths of Aging was written to take the same ideas in *Perfect Body* to a broader audience, and in doing so, contribute to improving the lives of even more people. As I faced the realities of aging, I saw that my family, friends, and acquaintances and the society around me need the benefits of better nutrition and healthier lifestyle more than ever before.

A Plan for
OVERCOMING
the Myths

Most of us want to be healthy, but we are not ready, willing, or even interested in making big sacrifices in our lifestyles. We try dieting, and it might help us in the short-term, but we soon drift away from the discipline we enforce upon ourselves because it is just not natural to us. So now imagine the possibility of living solely on meals that consist of 100% fresh, raw, organic fruits and veggies, 100% of the time. It sounds difficult, doesn't it?

We want our lives to be filled with possibilities, variety, and maybe a little decadence. This is exactly why this plan for *Overcoming The Myths Of Aging* was created—the *Overcoming the Myths* (OTM) plan. The OTM plan will help you find and maintain the levels of good nutrition, fitness, and positive attitude that fit your lifestyle, and it also helps you progress toward your goals for losing weight, looking great and leading a happier and healthier life. The OTM plan has three components: food, exercise, and mind. First let's focus on the foundation of the OTM plan—good nutrition. Here's how it works. The OTM plan is a tool to add more nutrients to your meals. Unlike diets, this plan is not about stopping yourself from enjoying what you love, but about helping you make healthy choices so you can have the energy to really enjoy your life.

The OTM plan builds upon the research and experience that is the basis for my book, *Perfect Body*. It seeks to eliminate the negative effects of toxicity that are the foundation of many of the diseases, such as high cholesterol and high blood pressure, that are common among our generation. The OTM plan also takes direct steps to curb the cycle of malnutrition that is caused by eating the junk food so prevalent in today's society, so that our bodies get the nutrition they crave and we end up eating less without feeling hungry. Later in the book, we will examine the linkages between what we eat, toxicity and malnutrition, and the myths of aging in more detail so that you can judge for yourself whether the OTM plan is right for you.

You Are Your Body's Worst Enemy

The United States is the most overfed and undernourished society in the world. Getting proper nutrients is the key ingredient to staying healthy. The reason I use the food program underlying the OTM plan as my guideline is because it is based on physiology—how your body works. Eating food based on how your body breaks down, stores, and uses nutrients, makes sense naturally. Above all, this food plan has worked for me personally to get and stay healthy for over 30 years. It has also worked for the people that I have consulted with for over the past 20 years. Using this program, my clients have overcome cancer, heart disease, diabetes, asthma, and many other diseases. They have lower cholesterol, lower blood pressure, and much more energy overall. They lose weight, look better, and feel better.

At the heart of the OTM Plan is the concept of "enhancing" and "compromising" foods. Enhancing foods are foods that deliver the maximum nutritional value to your body. They are easy to digest, and eating them adds to your overall energy and health. In the OTM plan, enhancing foods are fresh, raw, organic fruits and vegetables. This plan introduces ways to add more of these foods to your life. With the OTM plan, enhancing foods will account for the majority of the food you eat. You will learn how to use enhancing foods to maximize positive nutritional impact from meals and snacks, and how to balance enhancing foods with compromising foods so you do not feel like you are making the sacrifices that are the downside of common diet plans.

Compromising foods are foods that can introduce toxicity into your body or foods that you consume that do not nourish your body effectively, thereby encouraging your body to continue to be hungry and leading you to eat more to meet that desire. The

OTM plan helps you manage how much of these compromising foods you eat so that you get the maximum enjoyment from compromising foods while cutting down their negative effects on your health.

Compromising foods include animal products (the only dietary source of cholesterol), salt, sugar, cooked or processed foods (for example, foods that are roasted, steamed, fried, baked, dried, or boiled), saturated fats, and drugs (this includes alcohol, nicotine, caffeine, recreational, and over-the-counter drugs). If you check with the National Institute of Health, the American Heart Association, the American Cancer Association, the National Cancer Institute, the American Diabetes Association, and the Center for Disease Control and Prevention, they'll confirm that overindulgence in any one of the above compromising foods or substances can and will negatively affect your health.

Does being on the OTM plan mean you can no longer eat "comfort foods"? No! You can eat the foods you love on the OTM PLAN, and you will learn how to eat these foods with minimum negative consequences and maximum pleasure.

The OTM plan is focused on how much and how often you add enhancing foods to your meals. To manage the OTM plan, you will learn about a points-based framework that you can use on a daily or weekly basis to help you keep track of your nutritious meals and encourage you to introduce more nutritious foods into your lifestyle. There are several phases in the plan, so it can work for everyone and each person can approach the plan at his or her own pace and comfort level.

"The OTM plan is about winning."

In the OTM Food chapter later in the book, you will find more details on the points system and tips on how to use it to enhance your life.

Always keep in mind as you read through this book that the OTM plan is about winning. Even if you only add a couple of life-enhancing meals to your diet per week, you have increased your nutrients by a certain percentage and also improved your health. This is a plan about how much good stuff you can introduce into our lives. At any phase and any level in the OTM plan, you are helping yourself to lose weight, look great, and lead a happier and healthier life.

Adding Energy to Your Life

The positive effects of exercise are critical to defying the myths of aging and are a core part of the OTM plan. The established medical community reinforces the fact that physical exercise should be incorporated into plans for reducing the risk of heart disease, diabetes, cancer, stroke, and Alzheimer's disease. The OTM plan includes regular exercise along with the change to a more healthy diet.

OTM plan exercise is up to you. What is important is that you include a pattern of regular physical exercise into your daily life. You have plenty of opportunities for exercise throughout the day. Simple things like using the stairs instead of an elevator when possible, taking a walk at lunch, and taking small stretch breaks are easy ways to work more exercise into your day.

Physical movement delivers more oxygen and nutrients to your cells, giving you more energy and keeping you healthier. You will incorporate more beneficial exercise into your life through the OTM plan in a phased approach similar to the approach used to increase your consumption of nutritious foods. The OTM plan starts at a level that is comfortable for each individual and builds from there. Suggestions for OTM plan exercise routines are included later in the book.

Like the OTM plan for food, exercise should be something that you can enjoy and keep as an integral part of your healthy lifestyle. In the OTM plan, exercise starts with finding things you love to do and doing them. The key here is enjoyment. Exercise is supposed to be fun, so don't make it a chore. Playing sports, dancing, climbing, swimming, and running with your dog are just a few examples of fun exercises. Discover what fun is for you—what makes your body feel great—and then build your exercise plan around those activities. Exercise is physical movement for the purpose of making your body stronger, and you can do that during your workweek and while you play.

Growing Older, Never Old

Your beliefs about aging determine your attitude, emotions, self-appreciation, and your relationships with others as you grow older. I love the quote from George Burns about growing older, but never old. That is a fundamental principle behind the OTM plan. You understand that you are aging, and what the OTM plan helps you to understand is just how rich, fun, and fulfilling these years can be.

In combination with improved health and energy levels that the food and exercise portions of the OTM plan provide, the mind aspect of the OTM plan will help you change the disempowering beliefs that cause you to buy into the myths of aging. Aligning the mind and body is extremely powerful. The OTM plan helps you take control of your beliefs and create a positive dynamic that will help you lose weight, look great, and live a happier and healthier life.

"We don't have to buy into beliefs that promote the aging myths."

Your beliefs, in general, are based on information that you assemble throughout your life experiences. Family, friends, teachers, religion, society, medical associations, science, and the media can influence much of your beliefs. Most of your beliefs were formed when you were very young—much too young to be able to discern whether the beliefs were healthy, destructive or even real.

Over the years those beliefs have been shaped or reinforced by our social and cultural environments. Today, most of your beliefs about aging are also influenced by marketing and advertising programs whose sole purpose is to sell products, services, movies, music, and drugs.

The good news is you don't have to buy into a framework of beliefs that promote the aging myths. You can get the correct information; change your beliefs; and go on to live a happier, healthier, and more powerful life. Get it, believe it, live it! The point here is that it is your decision. The OTM plan will help you to identify the beliefs that are disempowering you, and help you create a framework to combat the aging myths.

In the chapter on Mind, you will create core beliefs that you will use as part of the OTM plan to take away the false power of the aging myths. You will do exercises for the mind and practice positive self-talk so that you can reinforce the progress you will be making toward a happier and healthier life. These mind exercises will become part of your personal OTM plan as a complement to and motivation behind your food and physical exercise tools for losing weight, looking great, and living a happier and healthier life.

You will take control and not let yourself be stopped by the myths of aging. You have invested far too much energy and emotion into your life to let it be guided by someone else's ideas. You deserve to be happy and live the great life you have earned for yourself. The OTM plan will help you to live on purpose, laugh, and anticipate the wonderful life ahead of you.

Roe:
The concepts behind the OTM plan are just part of my lifestyle, but I wonder if this makes sense to someone reading it for the first time

Stephen:
Well I think it makes sense, but there are a couple of big hurdles.

Roe:
Like what?

Stephen:
Let's start with a diet of fresh, raw fruits and vegetables.

Roe:

It's second nature to me, but I know people might opt out because they think it will be too difficult to give up the compromising foods they love. That's why the OTM plan introduces a way to balance enhancing and compromising foods. Anything else?

Stephen:

The idea that toxicity and malnutrition are at the foundation of many of our health issues seems hard to accept. It contradicts the common beliefs that our health issues are not really under our control.

Roe:

Again, maybe you need to start learning to question the conventional wisdom.

Stephen:

If I could get the information to see for myself how toxicity and malnutrition affect us, I might feel more confident that these are myths, and I would feel more energized about doing something to change it.

Roe:

The information is out there. It's available on several Web sites of noted research and medical associations. I'll put a list together in the resources section of the book.

Stephen:

That will help me, but what about the myths themselves? I think people will want to see how the OTM plan addresses each aging myth.

Roe:

Okay, that information is available as well. Let's get it, and then maybe you will start believing what you are learning, or start disbelieving what you think you know which is even more important with the myths. Once that happens, living it is easy.

THE SICK
Myth

My body is over 50 and I am not falling apart. On the other hand, I know people in their 30s who are already starting with the aches, pains, loss of energy, and diseases of aging.

I overheard a conversation between two women who were in their early 40s talking about their aches and pains, what medications they were on, and their latest doctor's visit. The conversation ended with one woman saying, "We have to just expect to feel worse as we get older." The other nodded with agreement.

Who said we have to feel worse as we get older? Well, of course, *they* said. Who are "they"? Society, the media, the medical and pharmaceutical industries, family, friends, the government, churches, schools? But are "they" right? Absolutely not!

Aging is not the cause of disease. If you look further into the research you will find a simpler and more believable cause—toxicity.

"You are the biggest cause of toxicity in your system. Or at least your diet is."

The more toxins you put into your body, the more your immune system has to work at getting rid of them. When you don't get rid of toxins they build up in your body's internal fluids. Then they proceed to invade and destroy your cells. I am going to share a little secret about what's coming: *you* are the biggest cause of toxicity in your system. Or at least your diet is. Here's why…

Your Cells

Let's start with your cells, because they are the foundation of your entire body. They are individual life forms, almost like microscopic human bodies. Just like your body, they contain miniature organs called organelles, which perform specific functions within the cells. These little organs help your cells take in oxygen, assimilate and digest nutrients, make protein and deliver it where needed, produce energy, secrete hormones, eliminate waste, and reproduce. Just like humans, cells come in different shapes and sizes. And also like humans, the ongoing health of a cell is determined by the state of its environment, what type of nutrients it gets, and its ability to eliminate waste.

Your Internal Environment

Your organ systems create an internal environment in which your cells can survive and function. Your internal environment is made up of the fluids within each of your cells and the fluid surrounding your cells. This fluid, your internal environment, is where all life processes occur. Oxygen and nutrients move into the cells from the fluid surrounding them, and wastes are excreted back into the same fluid.

In *Human Physiology*, the authors Vander, Sherman, and Lucino write about the relationship between the internal environment, the cells, and life: "A multicellular organism can survive only as long as it is able to maintain the composition of its internal environment in a state compatible with the survival of its individual cells."

This means that because your body is made up of individual cells, you can only be as healthy as your cells. If one of your cells is at risk, all of your cells are at risk because the same internal fluids feed them. Therefore, your health and ultimately your life depend upon the conditions of your internal environment.

STEPHEN ASKS:

What do you mean by toxic? I think we all know about the increase in pollution in our environment and traces of pollution in our foods. I don't think anybody is intentionally seeking out mercury-laden fish or purposely not washing their fruit to ingest extra pesticides.

According to the science of physiology, any substance that is not inherent, or natural, to the state of the internal environment is toxic or poisonous to your body. Toxins can enter your body through your lungs, skin, orifices, and even your mind (research in the area of psychoneuroimmunology conclusively shows that negative thoughts, situations, and people can affect your immune functions and cause a build up of toxicity in your body). Sometimes you don't have complete control over what goes into your body, especially through your lungs, but there are many toxins you can voluntarily eliminate.

The most common way, however, of poisoning your body is through your mouth. What you eat usually accounts for the majority of toxins you take into your body on a daily basis. Animal products (the only dietary source of cholesterol), salt, sugar, processed foods, cooked foods, saturated fats, chemicals (such as pesticides and fertilizers), and drugs (including alcohol, nicotine, caffeine, recreational, over-the-counter, and prescription) are primarily responsible for the advanced level of toxicity in your body's internal environment. These substances are not inherent (or natural) to the state of your internal environment; therefore, they are toxic. When used on a regular basis, they can and will add toxicity to your internal environment, create free radicals, destroy your cells, and eventually kill you.

Free Radicals

Your body is designed to react immediately to anything that

it feels is threatening your state of balance and health. This reaction is usually internal and sometimes not experienced by you consciously unless it becomes a problem.

If the body cannot get rid of a problem, it will adapt to it. In the process of trying to adapt to toxins, molecules will become unstable. I'm sure you have heard of these unstable molecules called free radicals. These free radicals embark on a survival mission—their survival, not yours. Free radicals are unstable because they are missing an electron, so they set out to capture the needed electron from other molecules to gain stability. They will attack other molecules and take the needed electron. The attacked molecule loses an electron and becomes a free radical itself, beginning a chain reaction. Free radical damage destroys your cells, and if your immune system doesn't step in to stop the attack, your body will die. Excessive, uncontrolled, free radical production seems to be a result of an immune system that is overworked because of toxicity and can no longer protect your body from harm.

STEPHEN ASKS:

Sounds pretty bleak to me. Our environment isn't getting any cleaner and now, in addition to the contaminants all around me, I discover what I have been eating is the major cause of my own toxicity. I wouldn't have imagined that eating meat, salt, sugar, and cooked foods could be so toxic. How do we manage to survive at all?

You can't expect everything that goes into your body to be 100% pure. That's why you have your immune system, especially your liver, to help you out. You need to use common sense and choose your poisons wisely and infrequently. Your immune system must be strong in order for you to be healthy, and you don't want to wear it out.

Why the Liver Is So Important

Your liver is an integral part of your immune functions. One of its major roles is to operate like a filter. It captures and then eliminates toxins. However, if there are too many toxins, or waste products, the liver becomes clogged and ineffective. If your liver cannot filter out the toxins, they recirculate through your blood destroying your cells in the process.

Remember, what affects one cell has an effect on all of your cells and puts your body at risk. A buildup of toxins can affect nervous system and mental function, leading to fatigue, depression, or anxiety. A buildup of toxins can cause allergies and skin reactions. Also, inadequate detoxification accelerates aging, which promotes the onset of degenerative diseases.

Even the most common and most deadly of the degenerative diseases in the United States today—heart attack, stroke, diabetes, and cancer (the Big Four)—are caused by toxicity and not by aging.

STEPHEN ASKS:

> *Okay. Let's say that I am open to the idea that toxicity is a source of disease and we can ward off disease if we keep our immune system healthy. I want to get past the generalities. How is toxicity the cause of the Big Four killer diseases you mentioned, and how does what we eat have a direct effect on those diseases? Most importantly, why aren't we hearing about this from more sources?*

Times are changing and so is Western medicine. When I began my research in the mid 1970s, there was little to no information on nutrition. Health food stores were beginning to emerge, but all they sold were supplements and a few books, mostly on fad diets. Western medicine and the agencies that supported traditional medicine were focused on finding cures through drugs. Staying healthy and preventing disease was not a common topic. Now, 30 years later, things have changed. Western medicine is looking more to lifestyle changes to prevent disease. Nutrition, exercise, and stress reduction are emphasized as a plan to get healthy and stay healthy.

Today there is much more information available to us about the importance of changing our diet and lifestyle from the American Heart Association, the American Medical Association, the National Institute of Health, and the Center for Disease Control and Prevention. Unfortunately most people wait until after they get hit with one of the Big Four to start changing their diet and lifestyle.

Heart Attack

Coronary attacks, commonly called heart attacks, result from a blood vessel disease in the heart. The American Heart Association states that coronary heart disease is the single leading cause of death in America affecting 1 in 5 adults.

A heart attack occurs when the blood supply to part of your heart is severely reduced or stopped. Blood flow is impeded when one of the coronary arteries that supplies blood to the heart muscles is blocked, usually from the buildup of plaque in the arteries.

Remember, the blood delivers oxygen to your cells. If your heart is not getting enough blood, then the cells in your heart are not getting enough oxygen, causing them to die. When enough cells die, you have a heart attack.

The most common cause of coronary heart disease is atherosclerosis.

Atherosclerosis

According to the American Medical Association, atherosclerosis is the primary cause of heart attacks and strokes!

The American Heart Association describes atherosclerosis as a slow, complex disease that starts in childhood and often progresses as people grow older. In some people, depending on the lifestyle, the rapid progression can start in their thirties. Three proven causes of damage to the arterial wall are elevated levels of cholesterol and triglyceride (fat) in the blood; high blood pressure; and tobacco smoke.

Atherosclerosis comes from the Greek words *athero*, meaning gruel or paste, and *sklerosis* meaning hardening. It involves deposits of fatty substances, cholesterol, cellular waste products, calcium, and other toxic substances in the inner lining of an artery. This buildup is called plaque. It usually affects large and medium-sized arteries.

Plaque deposits might build up enough to significantly reduce the blood's flow through an artery. They can also become fragile and rupture. Plaque deposits that rupture form blood clots that can block blood flow or break off and travel to another part of the body. If either happens, and a blood clot blocks a blood vessel that feeds the heart, it causes a heart attack. If it blocks a blood vessel that feeds the brain, it causes a stroke.

Stroke

Stroke is a cardiovascular disease that affects the blood vessels supplying blood to the brain.

According to the American Heart Association, stroke is the third-largest cause of death, ranking behind "diseases of the heart" and all forms of cancer. Stroke is a leading cause of serious, long-term disability in the United States.

A stroke occurs when a blood vessel bringing oxygen and nutrients to the brain bursts or is clogged by a blood clot or some other particle. Because of this rupture or blockage, part of the brain doesn't get the blood flow it needs. Deprived of oxygen, nerve cells in the affected area of the brain can't function and die within minutes. And when nerve cells can't function, the part of the body controlled by these cells can't function either. The devastating effects of stroke are often permanent.

The American Heart Association also states "high blood pressure is the number one modifiable risk factor for stroke."

High Blood Pressure

According to the American Heart Association, one out of three Americans, age 20 and older, have high blood pressure. Between 1993 to 2003, the death rate from high blood pressure increased nearly 30%. High blood pressure contributes to stroke, heart attacks, heart failure and kidney failure. It makes the heart work too hard causing possible damage to blood vessels. Damaged vessels that supply blood to your kidneys, your brain and other organs can cause these organs to become damaged too. High blood pressure often has no warning signs or symptoms and it can kill you. The higher your blood pressure, the greater your risk!

Healthy arteries are muscular and elastic. They stretch when the heart pumps blood through them. When the arteries become unhealthy, as in Atherosclerosis, they lose their elasticity and blood pressure increases. Arteries affected by Atherosclerosis are clogged and stiff. Also, external pressure to the arteries can raise blood pressure. Salt is one of the main contributors to high blood pressure. Salt produces edema, the retention of water in the body, and the trapped water puts additional pressure on the blood vessels. Fat is also a contributing factor because excess fat can put additional pressure on the arteries.

Stimulants in your diet are another contributor to high blood pressure. Coffee, black or green tea, chocolate, alcohol, salt, black pepper, drugs, supplements, etc., can contribute to negative changes in certain nerve impulses. These nerve impulses cause your arteries to dilate (become larger) or contract (become smaller). If these nerve impulses are not functioning properly, and cannot dilate, pressure builds in the artery walls.

An unhealthy cardio vascular system may also contribute to increased risk of high blood pressure. In the case when poor cardio vascular health causes the heart to beat faster, more pressure is created in the blood vessels.

Cancer

Cancer is the second leading cause of death in the United States, exceeded only by heart disease. One of every four deaths is from cancer.

According to the American Cancer Society, only about 5% to 10% of cancers are clearly hereditary; the majority of cancer is caused by cellular damage that occurs throughout our lifetime.

Any normal cell in the body might at some point undergo transformation into a malignant or cancer cell. Radiation, viruses, certain chemicals, and toxins can alter or activate various genes associated with cell growth, causing the cell to mutate into a cancer cell. A healthy immune system will seek out and destroy the abnormal cells; however, if your immune system is weak, the cells will multiply and can form tumors and/or spread throughout your entire body. Keeping your immune system and your cells healthy is an important factor in reducing cancer risk.

Diabetes

According to the American Diabetes Association, diabetes is a now an epidemic and a major public health threat. It is the sixth leading cause of death in this country and a major contributor to serious health problems such as heart disease, stroke, blindness, high blood pressure, kidney disease, and nontraumatic amputations and is a major risk factor for heart disease, stroke, and birth defects.

Types of Diabetes

There are several different forms of diabetes. Up to ten percent of people with diabetes have type 1, formerly known as "juvenile onset" or "insulin dependent" diabetes mellitus. Type 1 diabetes develops when the body's immune system destroys pancreatic beta cells, the only cells in the body that sense blood sugar and secrete the hormone insulin, which regulates blood sugar. This form of diabetes usually strikes children and young adults.

Type 2 diabetes begins with insulin resistance, a condition in which fat, muscle, and liver cells do not use insulin properly. At first, the pancreas keeps up with the added demand by producing more insulin. In time, however, it loses the ability to secrete enough insulin in response to meals. Type 2 diabetes accounts for about 90 percent of diabetes cases in the United States. It used to be most common in adults over age 40, but the National Institute of Health reports that children are now victims of type 2 diabetes. According to National Institute of Health, "high-fat, high-calorie diets and lack of exercise are probably the main reasons for the rising incidence of children with this disease."

Diabetes is strongly associated with obesity (more than 80 percent of people with type 2 diabetes are overweight). With the alarming increase in obesity in all ages and ethnic groups, the incidence of type 2 diabetes has also been rising nationwide.

Preventing the Big Four

Most of the problems relating to and causing the Big Four can be prevented, and the OTM plan is designed to help in their prevention. Let's first look at some of the major causes for these diseases, and then we'll look at prevention.

The primary cause of heart disease and stroke is atherosclerosis—a buildup of toxins in the artery walls. One proven reason for this buildup is having an excess of cholesterol in our blood.

The Role of Cholesterol

Your body needs cholesterol. In your skin, cholesterol is used to form vitamin D_3. In the outer layer of the skin, cholesterol helps minimize the evaporation of body water and also helps to make your skin waterproof. It is abundant in the nerve tissue and instrumental in your digestive process. These are just a few examples of the important roles cholesterol plays and, in fact, every cell in the body needs cholesterol. Some cells manufacture their own, but the majority of your body's cholesterol is manufactured in the liver.

Your liver sends cholesterol to cells that cannot make their own by way of low-density lipoproteins (LDLs), the main cholesterol carriers. The liver also sends out high-density lipoproteins (HDLs) to remove excess cholesterol from your cells. Your liver, in combination with the cholesterol receptors in your brain, creates cholesterol and then keeps it at a balanced level. Reports on cholesterol are confusing. According to the media, LDL is bad cholesterol and HDL is good. However, if the body didn't have LDLs, it would not be able to deliver cholesterol to the cells that did not make their own. Both LDLs and HDLs, functioning properly with the liver, are essential to your health.

What if the body produces too much cholesterol? A condition called genetic hypercholesterolemia is the excess production of cholesterol by the liver. This condition is rare. People with hypercholesterolemia, a genetic disease resulting in the lack of liver LDL receptors, usually die from atherosclerosis before age 20.

STEPHEN ASKS:

Well, cholesterol is an issue that has been pretty widely discussed, and one for which many people and products, such as cereal companies, claim to have solutions. First, how would my body get too much cholesterol if my liver is functioning properly and I have no signs of hypercholesterolemia? What do you suggest I do to reduce cholesterol?

The cereal companies say eating more fiber will reduce cholesterol. Should I go hunt down that box of high-fiber breakfast cereal I have had in the cupboard for the last few years? I know it's in there somewhere.

You can get too much cholesterol by eating animal products. Animal products include all meats, eggs, milk, cheese, yogurt, butter, gelatin, lard—all products of animal origin. Animals are the only dietary source of cholesterol.

The body's system for cholesterol production and recycling is thrown off balance when you eat animal products because your liver cannot accommodate the increase in LDL cholesterol. Since animal products are the only source of dietary cholesterol and science has clearly linked dietary cholesterol to atherosclerosis, it seems very clear that your ability to manage your consumption of animal products would have a direct effect on your health.

"Animals are the only dietary source of cholesterol."

Dietary cholesterol causes the liver and the cholesterol receptors in our brain to stop producing cholesterol and stop sending out HDLs to clean up the excess cholesterol in our blood. This excess cholesterol accumulates along the artery walls causing a buildup and the condition atherosclerosis. Reducing dietary cholesterol allows the liver to function properly and send out the appropriate amount of HDLs to clean up any built up cholesterol in the blood. When you stop eating animal products, the liver regains control of cholesterol activity and begins to dissolve atherosclerotic plaque. So the good news is that your body can recover from the habits of a lifetime. Eliminating or cutting back on animal products from your diet will help keep your liver in balance, eliminate cholesterol problems, and dramatically reduce your chances of having a heart attack or a stroke.

As far as fiber goes, eating healthy fiber in the form of fresh fruits and veggies is good for you but fiber is not the magic bullet for high cholesterol.

According to the American Heart Association, "when regularly eaten as part of a diet low in saturated fat and cholesterol, soluble fiber has been shown to help lower blood cholesterol. Foods high in soluble fiber include oat bran, oatmeal, beans, peas, rice bran, barley, citrus fruits, strawberries, and apple pulp." In fact, all fresh fruits and vegetables have soluble fiber.

According to the American Heart Association, soluble fiber is made up of sticky substances like gums and pectin, which form a gel-like substance in the presence of liquid. The gel binds with cholesterol and the bile acids in the small intestine and eliminates them from the body. Bile acids are made from the cholesterol that is stored in our blood, so more of your body's cholesterol is used up in replenishing the bile acids. This will rid of the body of some buildup, especially in the intestines; however, eating fiber will not cause the liver and cholesterol brain receptors to function properly. It is the lowering or eliminating of dietary cholesterol that will get the liver to produce the HDLs necessary to rid of the blood of excess cholesterol. That's why you'll notice on the side of those cereal boxes that the benefits of fiber always come along with a recommendation to lower cholesterol intake.

STEPHEN ASKS:

Beside keeping my cholesterol low and maybe getting a new boss, what can I do to prevent high blood pressure? High blood pressure is also a big contributor to heart disease and stroke, right? Doesn't age play a part in developing high blood pressure?

The American Heart Association states that high blood pressure can occur in children or adults, but it's more common among people over age 35. According to recent studies, aging alone is not responsible for high blood pressure.

However, it is has become a very common condition in our society based on our lifestyle. The problem is we allow our bodies to be filled with toxicity, unmanaged stress and relatively no physical moment. And, the longer we continue to live life this way (what we call aging) the worse it gets.

How to prevent or eliminate high blood pressure

According to the National Heart, Lung and Blood Institute of the National Institutes of Health, high blood pressure is a condition that most people have at some point in their lives due to unhealthy diet and lifestyles. However, in most cases high blood pressure is preventable and reversible.

You can take steps to prevent or eliminate high blood pressure – adopt a healthy diet, lose weight if you're overweight, limit salt, alcohol and other stimulants, exercise, manage your stress, and don't smoke.

I have talked about diet and the toxins that contribute to an unhealthy and stressed body and I want to point out that salt is not only one of the main contributors to high blood pressure, but one the most common toxic substances you put into your body. Trace amounts of natural salt in fresh fruits and vegetables enhance health, while added salt can destroy it. Salt dehydrates your body. Dehydration is dangerous from a health perspective and also not very flattering. Think about a raison, it was once a plump grape. What's missing is the water. Salt also interferes with your body chemistry by creating an imbalance in your salt/sugar levels. This imbalance creates unhealthy cravings. When you salt level is high, you crave sugar. If you indulge in sugar, your body craves salt.

You will find salt (sodium) in most of your processed, packaged and prepared foods. Avoid it as much as possible.

STEPHEN ASKS:

What about cancer and diabetes, the other half of the Big Four? Are atherosclerosis and cholesterol the issues behind cancer and diabetes as well?

Remember, degenerative diseases, or conditions that cause disease, are generally symptoms of toxicity in your body. If you have atherosclerosis and/or excess cholesterol, your body is toxic. The American Cancer Society and the American Diabetes Association agree and suggest that poor nutrition, excess fat, excess sugar, a diet high in animal products, and a stressful lifestyle (things that are toxic or not natural to your body) are the primary causes of cancer and diabetes.

We already talked about how animal products, fat, and stress are increasing the amount of toxicity in your body but, yes, there is more. Another common source of toxicity is sugar.

How Sugar Acts in the Body

First, let's look at the difference between sugar in fresh fruit and concentrated sugar, as found in dried fruit, cane sugar, and other products. Fresh fruit digests completely and does not have a harsh effect on your pancreas. Concentrated sugars, however, are the real problem.

When the body takes in any type of sugar (carbohydrates), the plasma (blood) glucose level rises and the pancreatic beta cells secrete insulin. This causes the target cells in plasma to respond to insulin and send a signal back to the liver to stop the production of glucose. If enough concentrated sugars such as processed sugar cane, dried fruits, and complex carbohydrates from breads and pasta are ingested, plasma glucose levels become too high causing the pancreas beta cells to produce more and more insulin and become overworked. When this happens, it starts the deterioration of the pancreas.

"Poor nutrition, excess fat, excess sugar, animal products, and a stressful lifestyle are the primary causes of cancer and diabetes."

The overindulgence in concentrated sugar and complex carbohydrates causes you to get fat. The fatter you get, the more toxicity you are carrying in your body and the more you force your pancreas and liver out of balance. More than 80% of all type 2 diabetics are overweight. And because America has an obesity epidemic, type 2 diabetes is on the rise, even in young children.

Maintaining a lean, healthy body with a diet of mostly fresh fruits and vegetables with little to no concentrated sugars and complex carbohydrates and a regular exercise program can prevent and eliminate type 2 diabetes and dramatically change how much insulin is required for type 1.

Lauren's Story

In October, 2005, I got a letter from a woman named Lauren who read my book, *Perfect Body*. She was diagnosed with type 1 diabetes when she was 13 years old. She is now 27. She was obese from around age 5 to 11, became anorexic for two years, and was then diagnosed with diabetes. Lauren had no history of diabetes in her family.

When Lauren started the program, her insulin intake was at 31 units per day. After three months on the raw diet that I recommended in *Perfect Body*, her insulin intake dropped to 17 units. Her three-month average blood glucose level was 90 (70–120 is the acceptable range), and her glycohemoglobin HbA1c test result was down to 5.0% (according to the American Diabetes Association, the normal range for a healthy person is 4-6%).

Her doctor was impressed with her progress. He was surprised and unable to explain why she could eat a fruit lunch and still keep her blood sugars below 50 without needing an injection. In a disbelieving way, he said that Lauren's pancreas might be responding to her diet by creating insulin and that it reminded him more of type 2 diabetes, but added that a misdiagnosis is highly unlikely and that children would rarely acquire type 2.

Interesting observation? Type 1 diabetics do not make their own insulin. We know, however, that most of the diabetes in young children today is type 2 because of obesity and lifestyle.

Lauren limited her diet to only fresh-squeezed organic orange juice and pure water for several weeks and then she did a few days of just water. This was an approach to detoxification that is part of the plan in *Perfect Body*. Her detox symptoms, that included dizziness and some vomiting, were intense but she stuck with the program. I suggested she ease up on the detox process and go back to eating fresh fruit and some leafy greens. She is still detoxing, but at a much slower rate and she is strong and determined. The last time I checked, Lauren's insulin intake was 4.5 units and decreasing. We are looking forward to the day when she is off insulin completely.

STEPHEN ASKS:

Roe, it seems pretty straightforward when you break it down to the basics. Why don't our doctors tell us about animal products and sugar and how our diets might be creating an unhealthy level of toxicity in our bodies? Do they not believe it? What are they waiting for?

They *do* tell us. However, most doctors don't get to people until after the symptoms set in or they've had their first heart attack or stroke. Western medicine is now becoming more focused on changing diet and lifestyle as a way to get and stay healthy. Reports from the National Institute of Health, the American Cancer Society, the American Diabetes Association, the American Heart Association, and many other Western medicine organizations agree that cutting down or cutting out animal products will help prevent or eliminate most degenerative diseases.

The American Cancer Society estimates that approximately 90% of all cancers are the result of environmental factors and lifestyle, and could be prevented. The American Cancer Society also suggests that diets high in fruits, vegetables, and fiber might reduce the incidence of most types of cancers.

> *"Approximately 90% of all cancers are the result of environmental factors and lifestyle, and could be prevented."*

The Centers for Disease Control and Prevention equates the increase in the number of cases of diabetes with the rise in obesity and suggests that maintaining healthy behavior such as controlling weight through nutrition and physical activity can help ease the burden of diabetes and might actually prevent its onset. Fighting obesity and getting physically fit is another area where the medical community is becoming increasingly vocal. They even suggest for type 1 diabetes that a change in diet and increase in exercise can lower the amount of insulin treatment needed.

Toxicity, Not Aging

The Sick Myth tells us that our age is the determinant factor in the onset of illnesses. Should we expect to see our health deteriorate? No. I am not buying it, and the evidence certainly doesn't make a compelling case. We might have all taxed our immune systems mightily over the years, but the good news is that your body knows how to recover—if you give it the chance. Science has proven and publicized that a sedentary lifestyle, along with a diet that contributes to toxicity, is the true cause of most disease.

Stephen:
Can it be that simple?

Roe:
Why does it have to be complicated? You said you were ready to disbelieve.

Stephen:
Are you saying that by cutting out foods that contribute toxicity to my system, I can eliminate disease?

Roe:
We are talking about aging myths. The information shows that the Big Four diseases have a basis in toxicity, not aging. By cutting back or eliminating the toxicity you introduce into your body, you are doing the best you can to prevent these diseases, and what I have seen and experienced shows me that it works.

Stephen:
But is this an all-or-nothing proposition? You said that what affects one cell affects all cells.

Roe:
I believe that in my case, and for many of the people I've helped that have had serious health issues, eliminating toxicity is the only path to regaining health. But the OTM plan is all about choice. For people without serious health issues, keeping their immune system healthier is a big win. Eating more nutritious foods and cutting down on foods that contribute to toxicity will improve your health.

STEPHEN'S PERSPECTIVE:

The more I learn about toxicity, the more I get it. Maybe I am the biggest factor in controlling my own health.

I read the recommendations of the noted medical associations regarding what to eat and what to avoid eating after a diagnosis of one of the Big Four. It amazes me that they only tell people how to change after their diagnosis instead of helping them to prevent the illness in the first place.

It was as if a plate of romaine lettuce posed a greater risk than the risk of having a debilitating stroke. What were they waiting for? Isn't it likely that foods that are better for you after a heart attack are also better for you before you have one? Sometimes I need to be hit on the head with a brick to get it, but not this time! This connection was so clear, why would I wait to have a stroke to reach a conclusion this obvious?

I don't know if I will be able to prevent these diseases entirely, but it seems reasonable that I will be better off than I would be by not trying at all. I end eating the same healthy foods if I just wait to have that massive heart attack, right? I think I'd rather do what I can now and skip the heart attack part!

THE FAT
Myth

You might think, "I have to expect to gain a few pounds as I get older." And for most of us, this is maybe true. But the myth is that age and fat are natural partners. It doesn't have to be so. You don't have to get fatter as you get older. You get fat because of how you eat and how you live. In reality, it has nothing to do with aging. Age is not a factor in storing fat. Contrary to conventional beliefs, aging does not lead to weight gain; however, the older you get, the more years you have of poor eating habits, and that means that each year you tend to accumulate more fat.

When you understand how your body gains and loses fat, you have a better chance of getting lean and staying that way.

STEPHEN ASKS:

If I am comfortable with how I look, why do you think fat is so bad for me? I mean, many of us are not that much overweight. What's the issue with sporting a little bit more weight than I did when I was in my twenties? Does it hurt me that much?

Why Is Excess Fat So Dangerous?

According to the CDC, obesity is a growing epidemic that's threatening the health of millions of Americans. According to the American Obesity Association, obesity affects more than one in four adults and one in five children.

If you are overweight, you are at an increased risk of the Big Four—heart disease, stroke, diabetes, and cancer. As mentioned, the Big Four are responsible for more than half of the deaths in the world today, and over 50% of all people who are diagnosed with one of the Big Four are obese (over 30% body fat).

In a study published August 24, 2006, in the *New England Journal of Medicine*, a sample size of over 500,000 men and women over age 50 were studied from 1995 to 2005. The study found that simply being overweight increased mortality rates from 20 to 40%, and the mortality rates of those who were obese increased two to three times over normal.

"Fat is killing you."

Fat cells not only store fat molecules but as these cells get bigger, they absorb other toxins that are in your bloodstream. The more fat you carry in your body, the more toxic you make your internal environment. Fat is killing you.

Because of America's problem with excess fat, the National Institute on Aging says that millions of overweight and obese baby boomers are on the fast track to becoming disabled senior citizens, a possibility that could have dire repercussions for them and for the nation's already overburdened nursing home system.

Public health officials have said for years that obesity increases the risk of diseases such as type 2 diabetes, heart disease, osteoarthritis, and cancer. Now a growing body of research suggests that being obese—30 or more pounds over a healthy weight—increases the chances of becoming disabled at a younger age and unable to perform tasks such as bathing or dressing.

Experts are scrambling to head off the problem. The Obesity Society and the American Society for Nutrition recently called for obese older adults to lose weight to avoid becoming disabled.

STEPHEN ASKS:

Okay, fat is bad and we are all adding too much weight. Then this is a straightforward issue. I should just stop eating fatty foods! If I just adopt a low-fat diet, I am done, right?

When you eat foods that contain mostly triglycerides (fats), here's what happens. In your intestines, fat gets broken down into its component parts, glycerol and fatty acids. These fatty acids go through many changes on their way to your bloodstream. Once in your blood, they are absorbed into your fat, muscle, and liver cells. When you eat more fat than your cells need, your body changes these fatty acids into fat molecules and stores them in your fat cells.

Some people believe that by avoiding fatty foods, they will stay slim. Not true. This is where they get into trouble because carbohydrates and, yes, even proteins can also be converted to fat molecules. Your body can convert glucose (from the carbohydrates) and amino acids (from the protein) into fat molecules and store them in your fat cells. Eating too much of any type of food—fats, carbohydrates, or proteins—can get you fat.

STEPHEN ASKS:

In addition to fatty foods, the information that anything can contribute to creating fat in my body is depressingly helpful. Now I know where the excess baggage I carry around came from—everything! What do I need to do to fight the fat?

The reason your body does this is to protect itself. In the

event of a disaster or a famine, your body has the ability to live off its own fat in order to survive. If you are fortunate enough to live where food is plentiful and if you have the resources to buy food, then there is no need to store food in your body.

Aside from psychological hunger, you feel hungry because your body is not being nourished. In order to maintain health, the body needs sufficient nutrients. When you're not getting the adequate amount of nutrients you need, the body wants more and more food. It will create appetite and desire for food until it is satiated. The more non-nutritious food you eat, the more you will want because your body insists on feeling hungry until its nutritional needs are met. If these nutritional needs are not met, shortly after you feel full, your stomach will expand to accommodate more food, your fat cells will expand to accommodate more fat, and you will continue to feel hungry. So you can see how this artificial appetite, created by malnutrition, keeps you eating more and getting fatter. One amazing fact is that fat cells do not multiply after puberty—as your body stores more fat, the number of fat cells remains the same. Each fat cell simply gets bigger!

If You Don't Desire It, You Won't Gain It

In order to lose fat, the first thing you want to do is lose your artificial appetite. You can do this by eating foods that nurture your body. Once you are accustomed to being satiated, your artificial appetite will disappear and you will feel hungry only when you need more nutrients.

The second condition for losing fat is using your stored fat for energy. You can do this by eating less than you need, allowing the body to break down the stored fat and use it for energy. Once you lose excess fat, you can prevent it from coming back by eating mostly foods that supply you with sufficient nutrients and only enough food to give you the energy you need to maintain a lean, healthy body.

STEPHEN ASKS:

It seems that the diet section is becoming the biggest section in the bookstore. There are countless diets. Protein diets. No protein diets. Grapefruit diets. Raw food diets. Mediterranean diets. Why are we still getting fat when there are so many different diets available?

Remember the importance of nutrients in your diet. If your body is not getting its nutrients, you will continue to feel hungry. Most diets don't work on two levels. First, they force you to eat in ways that are not natural to you and you eventually lose the discipline and regain all the weight. Second, because they do not provide you with the basic nutrients you need, you never feel satiated and you end up giving up. The OTM plan is not a diet. It is a plan designed to add more nutrients to your diet so that you can be leaner and healthier and stay that way.

You have complete control of what you put into your mouth and therefore complete control of how healthy you are. You can get rid of your excess fat and keep it off by changing what you feed yourself. And you can no longer blame your fat on aging.

Roe:

Do you understand why I think that adding fat is an aging myth?

Stephen:

It makes sense, but isn't it true that our metabolism changes as we grow older?

Roe:

Yes, it can happen, but that is usually because most people slow down or stop exercising or doing physical work as they get older. Older people who keep themselves fit do not have dramatic metabolic changes. Also, you should not eat more than your body needs to operate, if you do less exercise and less physical work, you need less food.

Stephen:

And if I eat more nutritious foods, I'll eat less because my body will help me by being less hungry?

Roe:

Exactly. Breaking the cycle of malnutrition or artificial appetite is important and will lead you to eat less naturally. Of course, you do need to avoid overeating and that also has a lot to do with your attitude and how you feel about yourself. The OTM plan addresses that aspect of your health as well.

Stephen:

Keeping active is also important, right?

Roe:

It certainly affects how much you need to eat, and sedentary lifestyles are definitely shown to contribute to obesity. This is also one of the aging myths—getting flabby. Getting fit and staying fit is the complement to a healthy diet when you think about losing weight and looking great.

STEPHEN'S PERSPECTIVE:

I have tried a few popular diets. Fit for Life. Atkins. The South Beach diet. The thing is, I never really followed or stuck with any of these diets, because the idea of a diet was so confining. I adopted a few aspects of these diets into my lifestyle, but over time I just lost the discipline.

Reading Roe's other books, I began to think about the concept of artificial appetite and malnutrition, and it made sense to me. We have all read recent books like Fast Food Nation or seen films like Super Size Me. We are gorging ourselves with empty calories. It made sense to me that if I took care to feed my body the right foods, I would probably feel less hungry. I sensed that what Roe was proposing in the OTM plan was about what to eat and how to eat, instead of being focused on what not to eat. I knew I could live with that idea much more easily.

THE FLABBY
Myth

We looked pretty good in those high school photos. When we see old pictures of ourselves with our children, we also notice how much more shapely our legs were and how much broader our shoulders and stronger our arms looked. Of course they did, we were younger, and now we're aging.

Bring on the next myth of aging—becoming flabby. The myth is that we are just not going to be as strong and toned as when we were younger. Let's put aside the fact that we have very convenient lives. We use the car to do all our errands. We take the elevator. We use moving walkways in malls and airports. Our nights at home are often spent parked comfortably in front of the television. As we grow older, the common belief is that our bodies are just naturally going to get a bit softer.

Wrong! Keeping fit and active is important to maintaining a healthy lifestyle. Regular movement and exercise will keep your muscles strong and looking great, and as long as you are exercising regularly, you can keep your body in terrific shape. Regular exercise is a pillar of the OTM plan and an important aging myth buster.

There is ample reason to stop believing that aging alone causes your muscles to sag, especially when there are people out there like Morjorie Newlin. The first time I saw Morjorie was on *The Oprah Winfrey Show*. She was behind the curtain so the audience couldn't see her. They put the camera on her abs and asked the audience how old she was. The show was about fabulous women over fifty and the audience couldn't believe she was even fifty years old. At the time of the show, Morjorie, a champion bodybuilder, was 86 years old. What's even more surprising is that she didn't begin to pump iron until 1992, at the age of 72, to ward off osteoporosis. In her first contest, she won the women's 40 and older category and has been winning trophies ever since. Morjorie's muscle tone and strength can be compared to someone one-third her age. When I spoke to Morjorie and asked her about getting flabby as we age, she laughed.

STEPHEN ASKS:

I'm impressed by Morjorie, but we don't all aspire to be champion bodybuilders. Bodybuilding can be a gateway to fame, happiness, and even a political career in California, but I just don't see myself on Muscle Beach. Are there other ways for us to tone up the flab?

All of our bodies are a little different. Some of us are long and lean with muscles that are better suited for long-duration sports and some of us have more dense muscles, more suited for power training and professional bodybuilding. However, all of us can train our bodies to be fit, lean (no excess body fat), and flexible with perfect posture, great bone density, and ideal muscle tone.

Aging alone does not cause your muscle and fitness level to plummet. Poor fitness is due to not using your muscles and not giving them the nutrients they need to function properly. It's not aging that creates flab, it is an unhealthy lifestyle and poor habits.

Use It or Lose It

Recently, I was in a serious accident and crushed the top portion of my tibia, a bone in my lower leg. Within a week, my muscles had begun to atrophy. My muscle tone was leaving me —my muscles were getting flabby. Why? Because in order for muscles to function properly, have strength, and hold definition, they must move.

A few days after surgery, I began to gently exercise my leg and I could see some changes, but it wasn't until I was able to walk that my muscle tone, definition, and strength really started to come back. Within two weeks of walking, my calf was back to normal.

If you don't move your muscles, you get flabby. Period. It has nothing to do with age. Look at children who spend all or most of their free time sitting in front of a television, playing video games, or working on a computer—their muscles are mush.

STEPHEN ASKS:

Honestly, having mush for muscles doesn't appeal to me either. I know I can buy into the idea of regular exercise and accept the fact that age should not stop me from doing that. So aside from better abs, what's the benefit from all the exercise?

Besides helping your muscles be strong and look great, exercise is highly recommended by the National Institue of Health, the Centers for Disease Control and Prevention, the American Heart Association, the American Cancer Society, American Diabetes Association, National Institutes of Health, and many other health-related organizations as a means to prevent heart disease, cancer, diabetes, and other degenerative diseases.

When you exercise regularly, you train your heart and lungs and the rest of your cardiopulmonary and cardiovascular systems to perform more efficiently. The more efficiently these systems perform, the healthier you are in general.

Studies done since the 1990s that have appeared in many scholarly journals such as the *Journal of the American Medical Association* and *The American Journal of Cardiology* have shown a lower risk of the Big Four (heart attack, stroke, diabetes, and cancer), Alzheimer's disease, and other degenerative diseases among people who engage in regular physical activity compared to those with a more sedentary lifestyle.

Put Your Heart Into It With Aerobic Exercise

According to the American College of Sports Medicine (ACSM), aerobic exercise is "any activity that uses large muscle groups, can be maintained continuously, and is rhythmic in nature." It is a type of exercise that overloads the heart and lungs, causing them to work harder than at rest and increasing the amount of oxygen-rich blood to your cells. The more oxygen that gets to your cells, the more energy you have.

The important idea behind aerobic exercise is to get up and get moving! Again, find something you enjoy doing that keeps your heart rate elevated (just slightly higher than your resting rate is a good place to start) for a continuous time period, at least 15 minutes, and do it at least three times a week. This will get you moving toward a healthier life and a fitter, more fabulous body.

The heart and lungs get stronger and work more efficiently the more you use them and the harder you work them.

Working Your Heart

During exercise, your heart is called on to work harder than it does when you are at rest. Your skeletal muscles require oxygen for energy production; therefore, your heart needs to get more oxygenated blood cells to these muscles quickly. Blood cells are redirected from other sources such as from smooth muscles to the skeletal muscles to accommodate demands. The American College of Sports Medicine statistics show that muscles receive about 21% of a person's blood flow when at rest. During strenuous exercise, that amount can increase to over 80%.

Our heart and lungs work fast and hard. The amount of blood pumped per heartbeat, or stroke volume, must increase to meet your body's demand for more energy. Your heart's efficiency depends on its cardiac output, or the number of beats it can handle each minute and the amount of blood pumped per beat.

Training the Heart

You can train your heart to be more efficient by slowly increasing the amount of exercise you do. The key word here is *slowly*. You need to go slowly and build up your strength and stamina so you do not cause any injuries. You can think of your body like you would an expensive sports car and train your heart the same way you would break in the engine of that new car—slowly and carefully.

The more you do consistently, the more you will be able to do. Marathon runners are a great example of this. The more they train, the more efficient their heart becomes and the longer they can run with less effort.

Fight the Flab With Resistance Training

Resistance training involves contracting your muscles to push or pull weight. It can be isometric (without movement) or isotonic (with movement) and done with free weights, weight machines, or our own body weight as in push-ups and pull-ups. In the case of isometrics, muscles are pushed against something fixed or against each other.

Resistance training has been shown to improve bone density and strength in the elderly. Recent studies of stroke victims over 50 years old have shown that resistance training improved extremity strength and reduced functional limitations.

Resistance training has also been shown to increase circulation and, in turn, increase oxygen to the cells.

Tony's Herniated Disc

Tony was in severe pain, and could hardly walk. He went to a top orthopedic surgeon, who told him he had a herniated disc and needed surgery immediately. I saw Tony before the date set for his surgery and explained that a herniated disc usually is caused by poor posture. I observed that Tony walked with his left foot turned out, causing his muscles to stay contracted. The constant contraction pulled on the left side of his lower back, putting pressure on his disc. This pressure caused the herniated disc.

Removing the herniated disc, which was nothing more than a painful symptom, would not solve the problem. The cause of his pain did not start with the herniated disc. The cause of his pain started with poor posture.

Tony's pelvis was extremely tight—he could barely move it. In his work as an orthodontist, he had developed the habit of improperly bending over his clients, and he was starting to develop kyphosis and a hypercurved neck. He was also 30 pounds overweight, which added more strain to his already sore back.

I worked with Tony to help him learn how to walk properly and how to sit, stand, and bend. He learned exercises and stretches to loosen up his pelvis and his back, and he lost more than 25 pounds. Tony skipped the surgery and instead learned to let go of years of bad posture habits. It was a difficult and slow process, but Tony did a great job.

If your back is weak, injured, or out of alignment, you will not be able to exercise properly. A strong and flexible back is very important—ask anyone who suffers from back pain. The spine supports the entire body and is the body's structural foundation, although we might not realize its importance until we experience problems in that area.

If your body is out of alignment, it will interfere with the performance of the muscles and skeleton. Many of us have back problems ranging from minor discomforts to chronic pain, and with the exception of a few accidents, most back problems start with poor posture.

If you are fortunate enough to have a functional spine, your primary concern should be to consciously keep it that way.

The OTM exercise plan is designed to help you get and maintain great posture and keep you strong, fit, and energetic. Awareness of your posture and a regular exercise program will also dramatically improve your health and vitality.

STEPHEN ASKS:

I'm traveling quite often, and I expect many of us will be too busy to hit the gym every day because of our jobs and families. What if you can't go to the gym, don't have time, or just plain hate going to the gym?

You don't have to go to a gym or even leave your home to get in great shape. In the chapter called "OTM Exercise", there are effective exercises you can do at home or on the road to create and maintain an extraordinary body. With a good aerobic and resistance-training program and good posture, you can stay lean, fit, and healthy for the rest of your life. Here are some simple examples of how you can fit more exercise into your busy life.

Busy Moms:

- Join the kids for bike rides or walks with the dog.

- Make soccer practice your workout time. Walk around the field, do sit-ups and push-ups, a few yoga exercises, or try jogging in place. Other soccer moms and dads might join you too.

- Turn that coffee klatch into a group exercise session. Maybe have the group pitch in to bring in a trainer or yoga instructor.

- Take an after-dinner walk with the whole family instead of heading straight for the TV.

Busy Executives:

- Always, always take the stairs to go a couple of floors up or down.

- Make meetings that move. Invite your coworker out for a walk when you have something to discuss. The movement might even spark creativity.

- Take a break at lunch and walk to your choice of restaurant or have your lunch in a park instead of at your desk.

- Get the company involved in a sport or activity. If the entire office is doing it, chances are the entire group will stick with it.

Busy Couples:

- Take a walk after dinner
- Make a gym date
- Plan weekends or vacations to include sports or physical activities
- Take up a common activity like bike riding or hiking
- Go dancing together
- Have more sex

Now you know it's not too late to get healthy and in shape, and maybe it's not too late for everything else.

Stephen:
I think most people know that exercise is good for them, but we are just not going to be as active as we were when we were young.

Roe:
That's where I see the myth taking control. We have many opportunities to add exercise to our lives.

Stephen:
But isn't it harder to stay with it as we age? I know I get tired faster than I used to, and I get sore in places I didn't even know I had places.

Roe:
It's harder. Mostly because our bodies are making us pay for our past behaviors. When we were younger, our immune systems were stronger and our bodies more resilient. We could counteract the compromises we made and still have the energy to be active. It's likely our current diets don't have the nutrition we need as well, so we are by definition left with less energy.

Stephen:
So how do we debunk the flabby myth if our past is catching up with us?

Roe:
The good news is we can do something to change the trend. That's why I shared the story of Morjorie Newlin becoming a champion bodybuilder at age 72. Age was not a barrier for her. As we add more nutritious food to our life, we'll feel the increase in energy we need to start exercising more.

Stephen:
Like everything else, it's staying with it that is the difficult part.

Roe:
Just as important in the OTM plan is making exercise fun. If people find a variety of ways to stay active and that they like, such as hiking, dancing, or gardening, they'll keep up with the exercise. The key is to focus on things we enjoy, start slowly, and build up gradually.

STEPHEN'S PERSPECTIVE:

Disbelieving this myth was a no-brainer for me. I have an active lifestyle and love to be outdoors. I do travel quite a bit, but even then I find that I can get some exercise in if I want to make the time for it. Most hotels now have workout rooms—although with my company's hotel spending guidelines these workout rooms are usually no more than hotel room sized! With or without the workout facility, at a minimum I can exercise in the room with push-ups, sit–ups, and more.

Upon reflection, I realize that I might be in better shape now than I was ten years ago. One reason is that I am much more disciplined about making time to exercise, and also because I have taken up hobbies I really enjoy, such as cycling and skiing. In fact, these days I can more easily afford both the time and equipment!

I could see that there are a lot of ways beside the gym to stay active and fit, and if changing our eating habits will increase our energy, I don't see any obstacle to busting this myth. In fact, I think I was on board already, and probably most of us could find something that increases our activity and makes us happy as well.

THE TOO LATE
Myth

How many of us believe that once we get to a certain age, whatever that age is, we won't be able to do, be, or have certain things? While we don't often make the connection consciously, most of us think aging is directly linked to limiting our choices. How many of us have heard, or—heaven forbid—said to ourselves, "I'm too old to...?"

Who says we can't learn a new dance step, become more athletic, start a new career, or be sexy? (We'll learn more about this last one in "The SEX Myth" chapter.)

By changing your life with the OTM plan, you are recapturing the energy to do whatever you want. Also, you can begin to shed the beliefs that limit how you engage in and enjoy the rest of your life.

It wasn't too late for Morjorie Newlin to have a great body. She was in her 70s when her doctor told her he was worried about her getting osteoporosis and recommended a weight-training program. If she believed it was too late for her, she wouldn't have gone on to become a champion bodybuilder in her 70s and continue to win competitions in her late 80s.

It also wasn't too late for Ed Latson to get his health back. He was 51 years old when I met him, and he said he was tired all the time.

Ed had been on a high blood pressure medication called Vasotec for nearly 12 years and, even with the prescribed medications, his blood pressure was 150/90 and sometimes higher. He had also been on antacids (including Pepcid) for more than 20 years because he had acute acid reflux. His condition was so bad that he had to sleep with pillows to prop him up so that the acid did not rise into his throat. He also had a precancerous condition in his esophagus because of all the excess caustic acid. He suffered from headaches—usually migraines—on a regular basis, for which he took Vicodin. He was usually anxious, so he took a daily dose of Paxil, an anti-anxiety medication.

Ed was a heart attack waiting to happen and, for the most part, a total toxic waste dump. At 6'3" and 259 pounds, he was 80 pounds overweight, his cholesterol was extremely high (over 200), and he was usually very agitated.

It took some time and convincing from his family, but Ed finally decided that he wanted to do something to improve his health. Given his condition, it was a big step for him to even believe something could be done to change the quality of his life, but the turning point was his decision to try.

I worked with Ed over a three-month period using the principals outlined in *Perfect Body*. Ed made serious changes to his diet.

Ed's Story

I was first contacted by Ed's daughter Deanna. She wanted me to work with Ed because she felt he urgently needed to change his very poor health. I met with Ed to discuss whether he was interested in making a change. At first he wasn't. His words were, "You'll never see me eating rabbit food." Without him believing in and committing to change, I knew nothing would happen. Deanna, however, believed so strongly that she convinced him—using her Italian charm (guilt!). She told her dad, with lots of tears, that she would never forgive him if he died before he saw his grandchildren. He agreed to do it for a month. I knew he would be hooked after seeing what a month of detoxification could do for his body. I was right.

Ed's diet was standard American fare, more than 90% cooked food and a lot of animal products, salt, sugar, and cooking oils. The first thing I did was outline a diet consisting of more than 90% raw, organic food—fresh fruit, green leafy salads, fresh vegetables, and some raw nuts and seeds. Within six months, he was eating more than 90% fruit.

He also bought a blood pressure cuff and took his blood presure every morning before he got out of bed and every evening. In a month, he'd lost 20 pounds, his blood pressure started to drop, he had very little acid reflux and fewer headaches.

At the beginning of the second month, he started weaning off his medications. This was a slow process, because going cold turkey could have put him in physical danger. The body does become addicted and dependent on such chemicals. He was taking two blood pressure medications, the acid reflux drug twice a day, Paxil every day, and Vicodin at least five or six times a week. He reduced his intake of the blood pressure pills and the antacids to once a day for a week then every other day for the second week and every third day for the third week. During this time, I was constantly monitoring his blood pressure and it was steadily dropping. Also, the acid reflux problems were gone, along with the headaches. After four weeks of the weaning process, he stopped the medication completely, except for the Paxil. His blood pressure was 110/70 with no medications.

This was just the beginning. After three months, he was totally off the Paxil and after six months, his weight was 179 pounds. He'd lost 80 pounds, his blood pressure averaged 115/54, he had more energy than he had in his twenties, and he was calm. He still is.

No more anxiety, no more headaches. I asked him to go to his family doctor for a complete physical and his doctor was shocked. He said that he "never saw such dramatic change resulting from diet." He also told Ed to "keep doing" whatever he was doing. His doctor said he was in "better than excellent health" and that his blood pressure and cholesterol were low. He had the "prostate of a 20-year-old."

Ed's body just needed the opportunity to get rid of the poisons especially from bad food and medications, and get into a clean and natural program. Ed says that now he has "freedom from illness and pills for the remainder of my life—the life that I never expected to have."

There are so many stories of people who reach for their dream regardless of age. They do not buy into the "too late" myth of aging. What do all these folks have in common? Their beliefs, their attitude, and their energy. If you let the other aging myths sap your strength and conviction, you will allow the "too late" myth to take over. Remember, these myths are related. When you believe that you will be powerless to stay healthy as you age, you will also come to believe that there is no change possible. When you accept the myths that as you age you become fatter and flabbier, you won't have the energy to tackle new projects or a new lifestyle.

STEPHEN ASKS:

I'm seeing the potential, but I'd like to keep a good grip on reality here. I am not twenty or even thirty-something anymore. Aren't there real limits to what I can or should be doing? You don't expect me to believe I can turn back the hands of the clock, do you?

How often have you heard or said to yourself that it's too late to try something new?

Frankly, I don't expect to win the 100-meter sprint at the 2010 Olympics, but I do believe that if I'd like to take up jogging, dance salsa, learn to play the piano, see the pyramids, or start a new business, there is nothing to stop me.

It's the common approach to aging that I fundamentally believe we can change, and that's not reversing time or defying the laws of physics. Really, it's not even that hard, and if there is any magic, it's the magic inside each one of us. Your body has an incredible ability to keep you healthy and energetic, if you let it do its magic.

The solution is about being healthy and having the energy to do all these great things and then believing that you can do them. You can do anything you set your mind to.

STEPHEN ASKS:

Maybe magic is a good way to describe these ideas. It seems too good to be true. That if we simply change our diet, we will find that all sorts of wonderful things will start happening to us. Is it diet alone?

Your mind is likewise a big a factor in beating the myths. There isn't a single aspect of life in which you can't find examples of how your beliefs and convictions result in tremendous achievements. The key to beating the myths is in believing that you can and the rest will follow.

In the OTM Mind aspect of the plan, you will establish core beliefs and see how these beliefs affect your attitude, your behavior, and how you live your life. You will do exercises to uncover negative, disempowering beliefs and change them to positive, empowering ones. And you will learn how positive self-talk can set you up for success in everything you attempt to do.

Take a minute to realize where you have arrived. You have accomplished much in your life. Perhaps you've raised a family, created a successful business, or built a career. The myths try to convince you that you are at the end of the line, when in reality the research shows that your body and your mind are ready for more. You are better prepared than ever to embark on new adventures, with the knowledge and experiences of a lifetime in your pocket.

Stephen:
Why is this Too Late myth a focus of the OTM plan?

Roe:
The OTM plan changes our lives in two fundamental ways: how we treat our bodies and how we think. One of the things I find most sad about the aging myths is this too late myth that keeps us from making the most of our lives—every day.

Stephen:
Isn't this just a question of discipline?

Roe:
How you think determines behavior and results. If you don't believe you can do anything you'd like to do, whether it's starting a new hobby, teaching, writing a book, changing careers, or starting a new business, it's just not going to happen. You need to believe in trying and believe in achieving in order to see results.

Stephen:
Then discipline doesn't enter into this?

Roe:
Discipline comes as a part of positive attitude. If you believe in going after something, you'll be disciplined in the pursuit.

Stephen:
But some people just seem more disciplined than others.

Roe:
Those people believe more than others. If you ask them, they'll tell you that they believe in what they are doing. You need to first adjust the way you think, and then it won't be about discipline. It will be about results. That's why the OTM plan is focused on winning—on taking actions you can believe and on being rewarded with positive results.

STEPHEN'S PERSPECTIVE:

Okay, so I can't say that I am really into a lot of the trendy psychology lifestyle books, and I told Roe that much of this makes me feel like I should burst out in a chorus of "Kumbaya". I wondered, is this stuff really part of beating the myths of aging?

I remembered my introduction to Roe's ideas in Perfect Body. When I first read her book, I didn't think I could do it. More precisely, I didn't think I would do it. Maybe that was my way of buying into the Too Late myth. I was choosing to settle into my known pattern of living and letting it create my life framework. Within my life framework, I resist change by becoming an expert at what does not fit in.

On the other hand, most of us have found ways to make our careers and families work whether things fit nicely or not. In my career, I expect it of myself to consider the available alternatives. I started thinking of applying this same approach to my personal life. I tried things I hadn't tried before and found some new interests that I enjoy. For me the trick was to remind myself to resist that Too Late myth every day. Maybe I could make my first response to something new be an enthusiastic YES. I can change my mind later if I want. I tried this with the OTM plan too. I asked questions, but I also looked for a way to make it work for me. I found a way, and it wasn't too late.

THE SEX
Myth

Sex. What a great subject for the myths!

When I decided to get a Ph.D. after getting my master's in the fields of health and communication, I was most drawn to the subject of human sexuality. I knew that a Ph.D. required lots of time invested in study and research. I figured if I was going to spend that much time on something, I might as well do it in a field I found fascinating, interesting, and fun.

It's important to understand that you are never, and I say this with great emphasis, *never* too old to have sex. Think about it. Now that you know—by following the simple principles of good nutrition, exercise, and positive change—that you can beat the myths to have a great body, wonderful health, and a happier and more successful life at any age, you can certainly have great sex. And why shouldn't you?

Sex is a part of who you are. Your sexuality is part of your whole package. If you cut this part of your being off, you stop being who you are.

STEPHEN ASKS:

As much as I hate the idea of it, isn't there a certain point where our attention to and desire for sex diminishes? Doesn't aging bring with it a loss of a sex drive?

As human animals, we are programmed to reproduce. When our body reaches puberty, our sex drive kicks in, and is incredibly powerful. In fact, and I'm sure you remember, sometimes the only thing we could think about was sex. As you get older, and your body is no longer gearing up for reproduction, your sex drive will change from constantly on to a more healthy level of sexual desire, as long as you keep yourself healthy both physically and mentally.

Your Brain Is Sexy

Your brain is your most important sex organ. If anything is stopping you from having a great sex life, it is what you think and what you believe. Remember, what you think and what you believe determines your attitude. Conversely, if there is any place to start changing the sex myth, it's in how you think about love, romance, partnership, and sex.

Are we ever too old to have fun, playful, loving, and romantic relationships? No! These are the best relationships as well as the sexiest. But what usually happens after we fall in love? Most of the time, we start our relationships being attentive, romantic, and having sex. Then what happens? We start to take each other for granted. We forget about the love, the connection, and even the sex. We settle into a relationship based on day-to-day responsibilities—working, taking care of the house, raising our kids, etc. But what happens to the relationship? Without any loving attention, the relationship grows stale. So we end up blaming our responsibilities, blaming each other, or placing blame on getting older because we are not living the relationship we had when we were younger.

STEPHEN ASKS:

We are not carefree teenagers anymore. We have stressful jobs, families to take care of, and often parents and extended family to care for as well. We are busy. That's just a fact. How can we expect these demands not to have an effect on our relationships and our sex lives?

Yes, we are busy. Most of us have careers and family responsibilities that take up a lot of our time. This is why you need to set priorities. If you want a great relationship, you have to make time for it. Balance in your life is an important part of staying healthy and being capable of dealing with day-to-day stressors. If you have a career that requires you to work late, make at least one night a week a special date night. If you still have young children at home, get a sitter.

Great relationships don't require a lot of time, just quality time. When you are together, consciously make time to have venting sessions to whine, complain, and curse about work, responsibility, anything, or anybody (except each other). Remember, you are on the same team. After the venting sessions, talk about what you love and appreciate about each other and how grateful you are to be in each other's lives. Be romantic and loving and sexual. This will keep your relationship fabulous.

If you don't feel loving and appreciative toward your partner, you are either in the wrong relationship or you don't feel that way about yourself.

The basic ingredients for great relationships come from within you. When you know, love, and care for yourself and when you are happy and playful, you establish a foundation to build playful, loving, and caring relationships with others.

STEPHEN ASKS:

Aside from the time a great relationship takes, isn't there just the plain truth to face? In my mind's eye, I may still see myself as sexy, but when I look into that mirror each morning what I see is older. How can I feel sexy?

When you don't feel sexy, you are focusing on something, like age or looks, that is outside of who you are as a person. Being sexy is a decision. Being sexy is an attitude. When you are playful and really enjoy the sensuous side of who you are, you are sexy.

This sexiness has nothing to do with looks or age, but it definitely has to do with attitude. That attitude comes from knowing yourself, loving yourself, and having a positive self-image.

Knowing Yourself Is the Foundation of a Great Love Life

Self-knowledge is about knowing your body; how to take care of it; and how to identify its needs, wants, and sources of enjoyment. What makes you feel good? What gives you energy? What depletes your energy? What makes you happy or sad?

Getting to know how your own body best operates is part of creating the foundation for a great love life. Once you have a connection with your mind and body, you can begin to understand and express what will make for a more romantic, playful, and sexual relationship. You will also be better able to ensure you are physically and mentally ready to participate and enjoy the relationship more fully. Age doesn't prevent you from knowing yourself—if anything you should be better at it!

Loving Yourself Makes It Easy

Self-love includes self-respect, self-esteem (your opinion of your contributions), self-worth (how much you value your contributions), and self-protection (caring about yourself and protecting yourself from pain and harm).

"It is not aging that defines you or your image; it's your beliefs that define you"

Loving and respecting yourself leads to more happiness, better health, and greater success, as well as an enhanced ability to love and respect others. When you love yourself, you take responsibility for your actions and protect yourself from harm—including protecting yourself from getting sick, fat, and flabby. The ability to love and protect yourself is not age-related.

When you love yourself, you choose to be with people who love you and demonstrate that love. You also choose to be with people who love themselves and are therefore joyful.

When you act in a kind, loving, respectful, and responsible manner toward yourself, you send a very powerful message to your subconscious that you are worthwhile. You are more confident and more willing to connect with your partner.

Positive Self-Image Makes It Possible

Loving yourself is the basis for a positive self-image. Your self-image is how you see yourself. Working on establishing powerful core beliefs about yourself is the first step to a great self-image.

You might know someone with a great body who thinks he or she is too fat or a beautiful woman who believes she is ugly. You probably think that they have issues. So when you look at yourself in the mirror and see a wrinkle or laugh line and you equate that with being less attractive, less desirable, or less sexy, then isn't that the same kind of issue?

"In 2005, over $10 billion was spent on cosmetic procedures in the United States and we still do not feel younger."

It is not aging that defines you or your image; it's your beliefs that define you. As a society, we spend an amazing amount of money on products and procedures to stop aging, and we never stop it. Over $10 billion was spent on cosmetic procedures in the United States alone in 2005. The sad fact is that after all that, we still do not feel younger. Why? Because we *aren't* younger and the myths exploit that fact as their weapon. Youth is part of life and being older is another part. One is not better or worse than the other.

Acceptance is the key. Have gratitude for still being above ground, ready for another great day, because if you stop getting older, you die.

Your positive self-image is independent of age. Age cannot stop you from living a healthy, fit, and active life. You can improve your physique, stamina, and looks and feel great about it. You can work with what you have or don't have and enhance or make the best of it. You can dress and decorate to express your personal style. Establishing positive core beliefs about yourself and creating your own personally attractive image is the fuel for better, more playful, and more passionate relationships.

Feeling Inadequate

Your body image additionally plays a critical part in your pleasure, especially in sexual pleasure. In addition to your beliefs, how you see yourself—whether accurate or not—will also determine how you are sexually (especially with a partner), the quality of partner you choose, and how much pleasure you allow yourself to have.

When you lose energy, gain weight, and/or start to buy into the myths of aging, your sex life can suffer. This can show up differently for men and women.

For men it usually is a performance issue. Men can feel inadequate and definitely not sexy. Many men use drugs like Viagra to help stimulate sex drive and performance. This, along with pursuing a younger partner, creates the illusion of being young again.

Women, on the other hand, lose sex drive. They feel inadequate when they don't look and feel young, thin, and beautiful. If they buy into the aging myths and compare themselves to young supermodels, they tend to fall very short.

Both men and women might take their partner's behavior personally and believe that their partner is no longer interested in them because they are getting old and losing their sex appeal.

Gaining energy and having a more fit body will make you feel better about yourself, no matter how old you are. Being positive and having a great attitude about life will keep you playful, fun to be around, and sexy.

Enjoying Yourself

It is important to allow yourself pleasure. When you take time for yourself to pamper yourself, do things you love to do, and be with people you enjoy, it builds your capacity for pleasure and increases your ability to accept pleasure. Your partner deserves this as well.

You need to love your body and take great pleasure in making it the best it can be – keeping it healthy and fit. Think our body as a gift, a temple, a piece of art. Have fun improving how you feel, enhancing how you look and decorating.

Age is not a limiting factor in allowing your mind and body to enjoy heightened emotional, sensual, and sexual pleasure. When you are playful and really enjoy the sensuous side of who you are, you are sexy. When you enjoy yourself, you can really enjoy and be sexy with your partner.

OTM Tips for Being a Great Sex Partner

- Develop a great self-image—know yourself, love yourself, and respect yourself.
- Know what gives you pleasure and tell your partner.
- Ask your partner what gives him or her pleasure.
- Have a strong desire to please your partner.
- Enjoy each other—be playful and romantic and laugh together.
- Be responsible to yourself and your partner about safe sex.

In the beginning of a relationship, turning someone on or getting turned on seems to come naturally. However, as the relationship continues, it's easy to forget to play with your partner and sex can become stale. If you follow these four steps, your sex life can become exciting, fun, and satisfying.

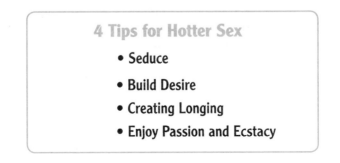

4 Tips for Hotter Sex

- **Seduce**
- **Build Desire**
- **Creating Longing**
- **Enjoy Passion and Ecstacy**

Seduce

The power of seduction is in the mind. Your beliefs about yourself and your attitude are your most powerful seduction tools. Your body and especially your senses will follow the lead of your thoughts and feelings. Form the intention in your mind and use your senses to gain your partner's interest and arouse his or her desire. Give yourself permission to be sensual and erotic with your partner. Look, talk, smell, taste, and touch. Smile! Flirt! Tease! Start with a look, a smile, a movement, or a touch and build slowly to more intense seduction. Sharing fantasies are wonderful for seduction. Seduction is a dance. Move forward. Move back. Most of all, enjoy the process.

Build Desire

Desire begins to move you from the mind into the body. Your senses play the key role, so make sure to take the time to use them. Keep the lights on and use your eyes, ears, nose, mouth, and skin.

Dress and undress for sex. Undress for you partner, slowly and intentionally. Watch your partner watch you. Dance. Watch videos together. Set the atmosphere with candles, soft music, and scents. Breathe in your partner's scents, sigh, engage in love talk, whisper, talk "dirty," sensually describe fantasies, touch, rub, bathe together, and massage each other. Do whatever looks, smells, tastes, sounds, and feels good that is sexy and safe. Be creative and use your imagination!

Create Longing

Take your time. Play, breathe, and create longing. Go slow. Allow your sexual desire to get so strong it is overwhelming. This might be easier in new relationship when there is novelty and more difficult with someone with whom you have history. However, the sexual rewards are greater with a committed partner and, if you are both willing to let go and move forward, the emotional bond between you will deepen and you will recreate passion in your relationship.

Enjoy Passion and Ecstasy

Building passion will allow the body to take over completely. The mind is quiet and the brain shuts off. You have the feeling of complete and total surrender. This type of ecstasy is all-encompassing—physical, mental, emotional, and spiritual.

OTM Plan for Creating More Intimacy and Mutual Pleasure

Don't rely on your partner to know more about your body and your pleasure than you do. You know your body intimately, and now it's time to share that wealth of information. Also, don't assume that you know what they like based on your own body. Everyone is different. Find out what makes them hot. These exercises are to help you learn more about your partner's body and for your partner to learn more about yours.

You can use the following exercise to reach a new level of intimacy, communication, and pleasure. There are no age or pleasure limitations.

Getting to Know Each Other

Here's an exercise on how you and your partner can get to know each other's sensual and sexual selves. Answer these questions honestly. You can do this as a verbal exercise by asking and answering the questions, or you both can write your answers down and then discuss them. You might even want to keep a journal to record your answers. It would be interesting to see in six months, a year, or five years if your answers are the same or very different.

1. What do you love, don't particularly like, and are neutral about sexually?
2. What turns you on visually, and what turns you off?
3. What sounds or words do you like to make or hear when you are being sexual?
4. What smells get you excited, and which ones give you a headache?

5. What tastes are yummy when you are sexual, and which ones don't taste good?

6. What flavors of foods, lotions, and oils would you enjoy using to enhance smell and taste?

7. How do you like being touched? What is too hard and too soft for you?

8. Where do you like being touched? Explore your entire body, and find all your hot spots.

9. What kind of movement do you like? What is too fast and too slow?

10. How do you want your partner to look, smell, and taste?

11. Do you like to share self-pleasure?

12. When do you like to fantasize about sex?

13. What types of fantasies turn you on?

14. Do you like to experiment with different kinds of fantasies?

15. Do you like to share fantasies?

16. Do you like to act out some fantasies?

Ideas for Sharing Fantasies

Fantasies are wonderful ways of exploring and communicating your sexual and sensual self. Sharing fantasies with a partner can be very hot and intimate. Sharing fantasies is a powerful tool to:

• Define and clarify your feelings

• Enrich your sexual experiences together

• Enhance intimacy and trust

Play with fantasies with your partner. Share some of the fantasy exercises below, or make up some new ones.

Bathing With Your Partner

Bathing with a partner is sensuous and erotic. As you bathe your partner, let each step of the process teach you something new about them. When it is your turn to be bathed, give yourself permission to totally let go, relax, and be taken care of. Here are a few tips that can make bathing together more adventurous and enjoyable:

- Before your partner arrives, create atmosphere. Remove from sight everything possible that says, "This is a bathroom."

- Redecorate to create an unusual environment. Flowers, candles, and music do wonders for transforming a bath into a magical experience. Drape lush towels or beautiful fabric over the toilet.

- If you are going to take a bath, you will have more room and enhance the atmosphere if you take down the shower curtain or remove the sliding doors.

- In the tub, one way to bathe your partner's upper body is to sit behind your partner so that his or her back rests upon your chest. Then reach around his/her body to wash and explore. This can be a very nurturing experience.

Sensuous Erotic Massage

Massage is all about pleasure. Whether you are massaging or being massaged, get into the sensual nature of the experience.

If you are giving the massage, try experimenting with different kinds of strokes. Combine them. Vary your pressure. Use your fingertips, hands, arms, elbows, eyelashes, and chest. Cherish the individual you are playing with. Ask your partner what he or she likes and doesn't like. Get feedback on pressure and types of touch. Don't use any lubrication on one part of the body. Next, apply some talc and savor the contrast. Wash your hands, dry them, and apply some warmed oil to another part of the body. Relish the difference. What does your partner like? Be creative and enjoy the pleasure of giving pleasure.

An Erotic Massage and Body-Mapping Exercise

This erotic massage serves two purposes. One, to give and receive pleasure and two, to help you and your partner create erotic maps of your bodies.

- Choose who will receive the first massage. Let's say it's you.
- Set aside 30 minutes for each massage.
- For the purpose of this exercise, let this be an erotic, non sexual massage. Remember, erotic means to arouse feelings of sexual desire, not necessarily to act on those feelings.

The first half of the massage is entirely under your direction. You will tell your partner exactly what you want and don't want.

- What kind of oil or lotion, if any, you prefer
- Where to start—toes, shoulders, face, or elsewhere
- The amount of pressure you want
- The kind of stroking you want
- When to add more oil, cream, or talc
- When to move to another area
- When to change stroking
- Whether or not to use feathers or other accessories

The second half of the massage is entirely under the direction of your partner. You just lay back and enjoy. Interjecting only if there is something you absolutely don't like or don't want.

After your massage, continue to relax for another 15 minutes, or however long it takes, while your partner draws your body map.

On a large sheet of paper, your partner will draw an outline of a body to represent your body and do the following:

- Circle the areas where you were most responsive and least responsive.
- Draw thick lines where you liked hard touch, thin lines for soft touch, and short strokes for feathery touch.
- Become totally creative and detailed and have fun.
- Put the drawing aside to share later.

Now it's time to switch. You give the massage.

When you are finished, compare maps and share your experience of how this exercise was for each of you.

- What did you learn about yourself and your partner?
- What did you learn about each other's sensual and erotic responses?
- What kinds of touching do each of you like the best?
- How accurate were you in drawing your partner's body map?
- How accurate was your partner in drawing your map?
- Which type of massage was the easiest to give? To receive?
- Which was the most enjoyable, the hardest, the most relaxing?
- Which one would you like to repeat?
- Was it hard to give directions?
- Were either of you distracted by worrying about what the other was thinking, feeling, or experiencing?
- Did you both feel as though you were being listened to?
- Did you both feel safe? Nurtured? Pleasured?

Strengthening Your Sex Muscle

Kegel exercises are designed to strengthen and give you voluntary control over a muscle called the pubococcygeus muscle or PC for short. This muscle is the support muscle for the genitals in both men and women. There is a definite correlation between good tone in the PC muscle and orgasmic intensity. These exercises increase blood circulation in your genital area and increase your awareness of genital sensations. These exercises, called "kegels," will also add to your sexual responsiveness and increase control over your orgasm. If you're a woman who has sex with a male partner, it helps you grip his penis and increase pleasure for both of you. It also aids in restoring vaginal muscle tone following childbirth.

To find your PC muscle, head to the restroom and see if you can start and stop the flow of urine with your legs apart (without moving your legs together). The PC muscle is the one that stops the flow. If you don't find it the first time, try again the next time you need to urinate. Practice slow kegels by tightening the PC muscle and hold it as you did when you stopped the flow of urine for a slow count of three and then relax the muscle. Practice quick kegels by tightening and relaxing the PC muscle as rapidly as you can. At first it will feel like a flutter. You will gradually gain more control.

Kegel exercises are a must for great sexual pleasure.

A Word, or Several, About Safe Sex

At some point in your life, you might find yourself single and dating. Dating brings up the subject of sex. And sex leads me to the discussion of safe-sex practices to prevent sexually transmitted diseases. For the purpose of simplicity, I'll use the term STD to refer to all sexually transmitted diseases and infections, including HIV and AIDS.

Sex should be about pleasure and not fear. Fear is not the answer! However, it is up to you to protect yourself.

It's important to understand that people are human and humans make mistakes. Most people are not out to harm others, but sometimes they do anyway. The message is to be responsible for yourself and not to expect or depend on anyone else to be responsible for you, your health, or your life.

Basics for Risk Reduction

Approach safe sex from a place of empowerment. Remember, self-protection is part of self-love. If you choose to have sex, you can do so without fear of STDs, as long as you follow a few basic and simple guidelines:

- Do not exchange bodily fluids, specifically blood (this includes menstrual blood), semen, rectal, and vaginal fluids.
- Always use protection for vaginal, anal, and oral sex.

- Ask yourself these questions before having unprotected sexual activities with someone:
- Would you engage in any of these activities with this person, with out protection, if you knew they had one or more STDs, including HIV or AIDS?
- How can you know that they are free of infection?
- Would you bet your *life* on it?

Again, sex should be about pleasure and fun, not fear. All partners should come away from the experience feeling sexually satisfied as well as disease free. Practicing safe sex will help dissolve fear and heighten satisfaction and pleasure.

Talking about protection is extremely helpful and becomes easier with practice. Be honest about your feelings. If you are nervous, embarrassed, or inexperienced, you need to say so! It gives you room to experiment and gives an unspoken permission for your partner to be honest as well.

If a partner refuses to use, or allow you to use, protection, don't fight it. Do things that are low risk or better yet, find another partner, because any partner that does not respect your rights and desire for protection does not deserve to be intimate with you!

Debunking the Sex Myth

When you respect yourself, delight in who you are, believe that you are worthwhile and valuable, and care about protecting yourself from pain and harm, you can really love yourself.

Enjoying each other, loving and respecting each other, playing together, and nurturing romance are the foundations for a great and sexy relationship. There is no age limit. It's never too late for love, romance, partnership, and great sex.

Stephen:

Roe, I didn't quite expect this to be a focus of the OTM plan.

Roe:

You don't think there is an aging myth about sex, or you don't think you can do anything about it?

Stephen:

Yes, I think many people buy into the aging myth about sex. On the other hand, I also see romantic couples of all ages. I guess the feeling of being close or intimate with someone special is one of the best parts of life, and there is no reason to want to let it go.

Roe:

It might show itself differently over time, but sex and sexual attraction is a big part of who we are. Many times because of negative conditioning, lack of energy, lack of communication, and outside distractions, we forget how enjoyable being in love and being intimate can be.

Stephen:

So you believe I can have a fulfilling sex life my whole life? That being healthier and more energetic leads to a better love life?

Roe:

Yes. Your sex life will take shape in many different ways and might evolve over time, but I definitely know that if you take care of your body, establish positive beliefs, practice romance, and communicate, you will have a great sex life your whole life. That's why I included these suggestions and exercises in the chapter. In conjunction with debunking the other myths, these exercises will help you make the most of your love life and of the loving partner who makes your life so special.

Stephen:

Where do I sign up?

STEPHEN'S PERSPECTIVE:

This myth touches on some very tough issues about aging, and a tough one for me. In our society young equals good, and old is not so good (let's not say bad, shall we?) The myth is that you can't be sexy or have a great sex life because of aging. Worse yet, all the treatments and procedures cannot stop me from aging. It's no surprise that my wrinkles are having more influence over me than my mind.

So even when I become stronger, healthier, and more fit, I may still look in the mirror and see that I am older. I definitely need to go out and find a new mirror.

What I am beginning to understand with the OTM plan is that I should not stop trying; I just need to have another benchmark for measurement. I don't like the fact that I am getting older, but that is something I cannot do anything to stop. Aging might define the sex myth, but I am not going to buy into it defining me. I can still do things to establish and keep a positive self image. I still want to dress well, be well groomed, keep fit and in shape – do anything that makes me feel good about myself. I can also keep my relationship interesting and loving, just by paying a bit more attention. With a more positive self–image, I have a great foundation to feel more fun, be more romantic and maybe sexier too.

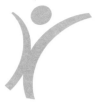

Stephen's Myths of Aging Summary Checklist:

✓ Toxicity is bad

✓ Malnutrition is bad

✓ Not moving is bad

✓ Stuck in a rut is bad

✓ No sex is VERY bad

I might be just a simple guy, but it seems like a good idea to take a closer look at this OTM plan thing Roe's talking about.

OTM
Food

Getting proper nutrients is the key ingredient for staying healthy. In fact, the fundamental physiological sources of cellular aging, in terms of the state of our health, are malnutrition and toxicity. We are the most overfed and undernourished society in the world.

"The fundamental sources of cellular aging are malnutrition and toxicity."

The reason I use this food program as my guideline is because it is based on physiology—how our body works. Eating food based on how our body breaks down, stores, and uses nutrients makes sense naturally. Above all, this food plan has worked for me personally to get and stay healthy for over 30 years. It has also worked for the people that I have consulted with for the past 20 years. Using this program, my clients have overcome cancer, heart disease, diabetes, asthma, and many other diseases. They have lower cholesterol, lower blood pressure, and overall much more energy. They lose weight, look better, and feel better.

Here you are, looking forward to the rest of your life. You want to truly live the life you've worked so hard to earn. If you want to be healthy, fit, positive, and sexually active, you have to have a plan to get there.

Does being on the OTM PLAN mean you can no longer eat comfort foods? The foods you love? No! You can eat comfort foods and, on the OTM PLAN, you will learn how to eat these foods with minimum negative consequences and maximum pleasure.

The OTM PLAN is not meant to be rigid, harsh, impossible, and unyielding. It is also not a diet. It is simply a recommendation for a healthier way of eating. The purpose of the plan is to help us beat the myths of aging and to lose weight, look great, and live a happier and healthier life.

What Is Malnutrition?

Malnutrition is a lack of healthy food in the diet or an excessive intake of unhealthy food, leading to physical harm.

When you eat food that is not easily digested and adds very little usable nutrients to your body, you are building up toxins and mutating or killing your cells. This creates diseases such as cancer, diabetes, obesity, heart disease—the list is endless. To add insult to injury, you can end up eating more empty calories because your body craves nutrients. The result is that you get fatter and have less energy, your body breaks down, and you age prematurely.

Nutrients and Health

Everything you feed your body is first broken down into nutrients and waste. Then the nutrients are transported to the cells by way of your internal fluids. According to physiologists, being physically healthy means that your body can maintain the functioning of all its systems to take in nutrients and eliminate waste.

Having physical health means that your internal environment is constantly kept free of waste and it supports the health of your individual cells. When you feed your body nutrients, your internal fluids stay in balance, your cells are fed, waste is properly eliminated, and your body is healthy.

The core issues are malnutrition and toxicity and the core solution is to eat healthfully.

Knowing the Essential Nutrients

Essential nutrients are energy sources your body needs to survive. These nutrients cannot be made by the body and therefore must be supplemented by food.

The primary essential nutrients are:

- pure water,
- carbohydrates (simple sugars),
- proteins (amino acids),
- fats, and
- trace minerals (such as calcium).

These nutrients are all created in plants. Plant food and especially fruits and leafy green vegetables are the original source of these essential nutrients. The nutrients in plants are complete and easy for your body to digest and assimilate. During digestion, you break down these nutrients into useable energy. Your body makes all other nutrients internally. That is why I advocate fruits and vegetables as the basis for the OTM plan.

Water

Water is your primary essential nutrient. Over 75% of your body is made up of water and water must constantly be replaced. Water is in every cell and involved in every function of the body. Going back to basic physiology, the condition of your body's internal environment, which is the fluid surrounding each of your cells, is what determines your body's state of health or disease. This fluid is mostly water and must be keep free of toxic waste. If this fluid dries up or becomes poisoned, your life is in serious danger. Therefore, your body must get sufficient water and that water must be pure. The quality and amount of the water in your body is primarily responsible for your state of health or disease.

Where Do You Get Your Water?

When you eat raw plant food, a large portion of your daily water requirement will be met by your food intake. Plant food is 80% water, this means, that in order for fruits and vegetables to be healthy, the water in your plant food must be free of pesticides and toxins, this is the major health reason to buy certified organic produce and to wash your produce with contaminant-free water.

You must also drink water because most of the time you cannot get all the water you require to stay healthy from your diet. Granted, water rich plant food is over 80% water but with exercise, heat, etc., you lose more water than you can replace with food. Unless of course you eat more food than you need and then you have the problem of excess fat. So eating more food to try to satisfy your daily water requirement is not a good solution. You must drink water.

The water that you drink must be pure or else you are doing more harm than good by flooding your body with toxic chemicals. Tap water, with chlorine, fluoride, radon, arsenic and other toxic chemicals, is not healthy. Filtered water, mineral water and spring water are not entirely free of chemicals. In fact, some bottled water tested worse than local tap water. Pure water is distilled. A vapor compression distillation process will purify water and make it healthier to drink. Another benefit of distilled water is that it leaches inorganic minerals rejected by the cells and tissues out of the body, adding to the purification of your internal environment.

Remember, water is going into your body as its primary nutrient and will make a major difference in the state of your health.

Protein

Your body makes some of the protein you need though recycling and reusing dead cells, and the rest can be supplied by plants in the form of amino acids. These amino acid chains are readily available to your body to build protein. If you eat animal protein, however, the protein is less readily available. Your body must break down the animal protein into amino acid chains and then rebuild them to usable protein. The process of converting animal protein to usable protein is very inefficient.

Protein Requirements

As an adult, how much protein do you really need? First of all, at what stage in your life did you need the most protein? When you were a baby and growing at a rapid speed! Healthy babies get their nutrients from mother's milk. Mother's milk contains approximately two percent protein at the start of lactation. It gradually tapers down to about one percent after six months and to less than one percent after one year. Almost 90 percent of mother's milk is water, less then one percent is fat, and the remainder is made up of carbohydrates — simple sugars. Plant food, especially fruit, has the same chemical breakdown as mother's milk. Young children, teenagers, and especially adults need much less protein than babies.

According to basic human physiology, once a body is weaned from mother's milk, amino acids from plant foods supply the human body with all of the essential nutrients it needs to fulfill its protein requirements.

Compromising Your Health

Your health can be compromised and your body malnourished by the following substances: animal products (the only dietary source of cholesterol), salt, sugar, cooked and processed foods (roasted, steamed, fried, baked, dried, stir-fried, heated, boiled, or fermented), saturated fats, chemicals (pesticides and fertilizers), and drugs (whether alcohol, nicotine, caffeine, recreational, over-the-counter, or prescription). According to the National Institutes of Health (NIH), the American Heart Association (AHA), the American Cancer Society (ACS), the National Cancer Institute (NCI), the American Diabetes Association (ADA), and the Centers for Disease Control and Prevention (CDC), overindulgence in any one of the above substances can and will compromise a person's health.

Compromising vs. Enhancing Foods

In general, when you compromise, you get less than you actually want. When something is enhancing, it adds to what you already have.

The food items, cooking processes, and drugs mentioned above are compromising foods. Consuming them gives you less of what you want. You end up with fewer nutrients, less overall energy, and less overall health. However, compromising also gets you some of what you want as well. The OTM plan is not about eliminating compromise; it's about making *good* compromises. We will explore this idea in more depth later, but the important thing to remember is that you have a choice. You can choose to create the right balance of enhancing and compromising foods for yourself.

Enhancing foods are fresh, raw, organic fruits and vegetables. Eating them adds to your overall energy and health. However, getting the maximum nutritional value out of these foods requires that you eat them by themselves, without any of the compromising foods.

Making Compromise Work

People eat compromising foods for fun and not to enhance their overall health. Your body, especially when you keep yourself healthy, can handle small amounts of compromising foods without any, or very little, negative effects. Eating a small amount of compromising foods, especially concentrated proteins like animal products, soy, nuts, and seeds and complex carbohydrates such as pasta, rice, and potatoes with a large green salad will give you the natural enzymes you need to help break down these foods.

The Ideal Way to Eat

If you want to get the most out of food, you must eat the enhancing foods alone as a separate meal or at least an hour before adding any foods from the compromising group. For example, eat a bowl of fresh grapes and nothing else. In an hour the grapes will have done their job, giving you the nutrients you need. It is also important not to eat anything compromising for at least an hour before eating fruit. So if you just had a piece of pizza, you should wait at least an hour before indulging in those grapes.

When eating fruit, a mono fruit meal is ideal. A mono meal means eating just one type of food at a meal; for example, have five peaches or 16 ounces of fresh-squeezed orange juice instead of a fruit salad or a smoothie. When eating a salad with more than just salad greens, ideally mix the salad greens with only one fruit or vegetable, such as avocados, and a very simple dressing like extra-virgin olive oil with fresh-squeezed juice from a lemon or orange.

Stephen:
Is the OTM food plan a 100% fresh, organic, raw fruit and vegetable diet?

Roe:
The basis of the food plan is fresh, raw, organic fruits and vegetables. Remember this is not a diet; it is a plan to increase the nutritious food in your diet in order to lose weight, look great, and live a happier and healthier life. By adding more enhancing foods to your life, you will break the cycle of malnutrition and toxicity that make the foundation of the aging myths.

Stephen:
Would you say adopting the OTM plan is a vegetarian or vegan diet then?

Roe:
I see the OTM plan differently. It is not about what you can't eat; it's about what you should eat more often. Many vegetarian or vegan diets also include compromising foods. Proteins, nuts, and flour, for instance. There is mixing and cooking which also compromises foods. These approaches focus on what to exclude. If it's not meat, then it is good for you. I know vegetarians that suffer from the same common health problems, because they are making compromises that introduce malnutrition and toxicity into their lives.

Stephen:
The vegetarians I know don't see it that way, although I have seen plenty of overweight vegetarians too.

Roe: *I am not against the concept of vegetarian lifestyles. What I believe is that you can also introduce compromising foods—along with malnutrition and toxicity—into any diet. It's the focus on good nutrition that I think is most important in the OTM plan.*

Stephen:
So does that mean I can eat my dry-aged, perfectly marbled, and deliciously grilled T-bone?

Roe:
I don't advocate it, but on the OTM plan you can choose to make that compromise. Just as eating a vegetarian burrito with beans and rice and sour cream would be a type of compromise. The point is to balance compromising foods in relation to enhancing foods, and make the majority of the food you eat enhancing.

Stephen:
You mean like skipping the baked potato and starting with a big green salad?

Roe:
Yes, and by making sure that you control the portions of your compromises.

Stephen:
Can I have blue cheese dressing on my salad too?

Roe: *Don't push it...*

STEPHEN'S PERSPECTIVE:

Don't worry—my first reaction was similar to the one you must be experiencing. This sounds really tough to do, right? Who could live on just raw fruits and vegetables? She must have me confused with Bugs Bunny.

There was no way the plan was going to work in my life. No cooking. No mixing. No wine. That was the deal breaker for me. There is probably a deal breaker or two in there for you too.

Eliminating toxicity is the key, so anything that is toxic is bad for you. However, I thought that less toxic had to be better than more toxic, and I knew that the healthier eating habits that I had already adopted had helped me keep fit and have more energy. Those eating habits included more than raw fruits and vegetables.

I serenely poured myself a generous glass of compromising wine and reviewed what I had gotten from OTM plan so far. I know that I can have a big impact on my health if I take steps to reduce toxicity in my body, and what I consume is the biggest influence on my body's level of toxins. If I eat good, nutritious foods as opposed to empty calories, my body will feel less need to eat. With exercise and healthy eating, I will lose weight, feel fitter, and have more energy. Ok, so far it seems on track.

I don't think it's too late for me to make changes that I really WANT to make. The more I understand about how to manage toxicity and nourishment, the better I will be able to craft an approach that will deliver the results I am seeking. However, I still have a lot of questions to cover first.

OTM
Food Q & A

Okay, Roe, But What About...

When people first hear about the OTM plan, they often ask about many of the same things in order to get the information they need to learn to disbelieve. We have been conditioned to think about our health and our diets in a certain way, and this conditioning contributes to promoting the aging myths. Stephen asked me all of these questions, and I am sure you would as well if we were talking about the OTM plan.

Q: What about the five food groups? Your plan seems contrary to the eating practices the food groups promote. I have been hearing about food groups since I was a kid. In fact, they are still teaching it in school. Aren't we supposed to get several servings from each group, each day?

A: Western medicine has been endorsing food requirements and food groups since the United States Department of Agriculture (USDA) developed them in 1894. Unfortunately, the agricultural community first wrote these standards with little attention to physiological requirements. Current U.S. dietary policies still reflect the basic design of the food guides from the early part of this century. However, there are many medical doctors and scientist who don't agree with the USDA.

Let's look at the requirements for meat and dairy. Our physiological nutritional requirements for protein are for amino acids—those found in plant food. Yet our food guidelines from the USDA have always included generous portions of animal proteins. In fact, in 1933 butter was in its own food group. In 1942, butter shared its food group with fortified margarine.

In talking about animal products in our government dietary guidelines, the Physicians Committee for Responsible Medicine (PCRM) states, "This element of food guides has persisted until the present time, due in part to the intensive lobbying efforts of the food industry, and despite evidence of the adverse health effects of such foods." Based on current scientific research on disease and its relationship to diet and lifestyle, the PCRM recommends a vegan diet.

Now let's look at our fat requirements. Back in the 1950s, research on cholesterol was linked to heart disease. This created much controversy about protein requirements and the meat and dairy industries were up in arms.

In 1968, while the data on fat and health remained ambiguous and the scientific community polarized, the deadlock was broken not by any new science, but by politicians. It was Senator George McGovern's bipartisan, nonlegislative Select Committee on Nutrition and Human Needs—and, to be precise, a handful of McGovern's staff members—that almost single-handedly changed nutritional policy in this country and initiated the process of turning the dietary fat hypothesis into dogma. The committee policy for low fat is based chiefly on the fact that fat, specifically the hard, saturated fat found primarily in meat and dairy products, elevates blood cholesterol levels. This in turn raises the likelihood that cholesterol will clog arteries, a condition known as atherosclerosis, which then increases risk of coronary artery disease, heart attack, and untimely death. Instead of taking animal products out of the nutritional requirements, the committee decided that *all* fat was a problem.

This policy of a low-fat and high-carbohydrate diet backfired and contributed to the progressive increase in obesity in our country until obesity is now a growing epidemic. Why? Instead of recommending a sound nutritional diet with simple sugar carbohydrates (fresh fruits and veggies), the guidelines promoted more complex carbs (bread, rice, and pasta), contributing to the obesity epidemic and increasing our risk of the Big Four—heart disease, stroke, diabetes, and cancer. As mentioned, the Big Four are responsible for more than half of the deaths in the world today and over 50% of all people who are diagnosed with one of the Big Four are obese.

Here's some more history:

In 1894, the USDA developed the first food composition tables and dietary standards for Americans. In 1916, the first daily food guides appeared in USDA publications, consisting of five food groups:

- milk and meat,
- cereals,
- vegetables and fruits,
- fats and fat foods, and
- sugars and sugary foods.

In 1933, through intense lobbing effects, food groups expanded to 12 with milk, dairy, and eggs earning their own category.

In 1941, the first Recommended Dietary Allowances were released by the Food and Nutrition Board of the National Academy of Sciences, including recommendations for calories and nine nutrients. In 1942, the "Basic Seven" food guide was released by the USDA. Milk still held its own, and meat and eggs were grouped together. This is when butter and fortified margarine shared a group—because it was hard to get butter during wartime.

In 1956, the seven food groups were condensed to the "Basic Four" in the USDA publication, *Essentials of an Adequate Diet*. Milk is still holding its own and meat and eggs are sharing their spotlight with beans and nuts.

In 1979, the USDA issued the "Hassle-Free Guide to a Better Diet" which added a fifth food group to the "Basic Four," to include fats, sweets, and alcohol and recommended moderation in their use. Sound healthy?

The first *Dietary Guidelines for Americans* was released in 1980 by the USDA and the Department of Health and Human Services and has been revised every five years since then.

The Food Guide Pyramid, introduced in 1992, encouraged the consumption of grains, vegetables, and fruits but continued to recommend two to three servings each day of foods from a dairy product group and from a meat group. Because of protests from the scientific community and intense lobbying efforts by the meat and dairy industries, the USDA turned the pyramid on its side and called it MyPyramid, with 12 different guides to choose from depending on your lifestyle.

According to the Harvard School of Public Health, "The new symbol doesn't convey enough information to help you make informed choices about your diet and long-term health. And it continues to recommend foods that aren't essential to good health, and might even be detrimental in the quantities included in MyPyramid."

Again we ask, who built the pyramid? "The USDA's MyPyramid also had many builders. Some are obvious—USDA scientists, nutrition experts, staff members, and consultants. Others aren't. Intense lobbying efforts from a variety of food industries also helped shape the pyramid," added the Harvard School of Public Health. The dairy industry gained a much larger piece of the new pyramid. Got milk? Got good lobbying.

Long answer, but as you can see much of the dietary information is not based on science but on lobbying efforts, government committees, and social and economic pressures. Look around this country and see the levels of toxicity, disease, and obesity, it's seems more valid to question these guidelines than to believe them.

Q: But don't we need some balance? How am I going to get my protein without meat or soy proteins?

A: All your essential nutrients—nutrients that you need to get from food sources that you can't make yourself—can come from plants. This includes protein. Remember the most efficient way for your body to get usable protein is through amino acids. Breaking down animal protein is inefficient at best. Animal protein comes with other problems, including cholesterol. You might choose to eat animal protein because you enjoy it, but you don't have to eat it because you need it.

Q: The protein diets seem to have been working, though. I lost weight on them and so have many of my friends. What's wrong with that approach?

A: These diets do create results. You do lose fat, but here is why. Your body normally uses glucose to obtain its energy. The glucose you need comes from the carbohydrates in your diet. When you eat a low-carb, high-protein diet without an adequate amount of glucose your body thinks it's starving, so it elevates the ketone levels in your blood. This process is called *ketosis* and is the basis for the protein diets. Prolonged ketosis, more than two weeks and sometimes less, can be dangerous as it can change the acidity of your blood beyond the level that your body can tolerate. This might eventually lead to serious damage to your liver and kidneys. So high protein diets can get rid of fat, but they can also make you very sick in the process. And because high-protein diets are high in cholesterol, they eventually clog your arteries. We are already seeing the health fallout from these protein diet programs in the newspapers, and I think we will see much more. Remember, The OTM plan is not a diet. We are talking about a plan for better health that includes reducing fat.

Q: I read an article that carbs are making a comeback in the wake of the protein diet backlash you mentioned. However, you see these as compromising foods. Why?

A: Simple sugar carbohydrates, such as those made by plants and found in fruit and vegetables, are life-enhancing. Like amino acids, these carbs are readily available during digestion and more easily used by the body. When I write about digestion, I am referring to the breakdown and chemical conversion of food into nutrients at the multicellular, cellular, and subcellular levels. Concentrated or complex carbs, including bread and pasta are more difficult to digest. Your body has to work harder to completely digest these complex carbs, and much of these partially digested carbs are routed into fat cells because the body naturally seeks the simpler compounds. They're what we call empty calories. These are definitely compromising foods!

Q: What about calcium? Isn't this particularly important to prevent osteoporosis?

A: Your body needs nutrients in order for your bones to function properly and meet your body's requirement for calcium. I had an accident that crushed a bone in my leg. After three weeks, the X-rays showed that my bone was already laying down the calcium it needed to repair itself. My doctor, Bill McGann in San Francisco, said that I was healing in one-third the normal time and that it was due to how I took care of myself.

Our bones have two special cell types that are the maintenance staff of the skeletal system—osteoclasts and osteoblasts. In a healthy body, there is no bone that is older than 20 years. How does that happen? Bones are being constantly rebuilt, and that helps maintain their strength and resilience. The osteoclasts dissolve old bones cells, and the osteoblasts follow along and rebuild them. Increasing toxicity in our body damages our bone's maintenance staff and that can lead to problems like osteoporosis.

A healthy body is good at recycling calcium. However, toxic foods can throw this healthy balance off. For example, increased protein and increased sodium triggers the body to release more calcium as waste. It's a double whammy. Toxic foods are hurting the bone cells that help manage the calcium-bone linkage, creating greater need for calcium.

There are good, enhancing sources of calcium in raw plant food. Plants survive by extracting elements from the soil. These elements include calcium and are readily available to us when we eat raw plant food. We also have a reusable calcium store in our bodies. By limiting toxic foods that deplete calcium, we allow our bodies to easily manage our calcium needs and we can get all the calcium we need from enhancing plant foods.

Q: Where do vitamin supplements fit into your plan? Can't I improve my health by loading up on vitamins?

A: Fresh, raw fruits and vegetables have the completely digestible vitamins and minerals we need to keep healthy. Loading up on supplements only causes the body to work harder digesting these concentrated pills, powders, and liquids. After they are digested, some of these supplements pass right though us without causing any problems; however, some of these supplements are toxic and only add to our toxicity level. I would not indulge in supplements to replace vitamins I could get from healthy fruits and vegetables.

Q: Vegetables and leafy greens are good for you, right? They are nutritious foods, so why does cooking them make them a compromising food?

A: Cooking destroys most food enzymes. Plant enzymes are proteins created in plants. These enzymes act as a catalyst to help speed up digestion. Because they are protein, they are sensitive to heat and are usually destroyed in the process of cooking.

Several studies have been conducted to show the effects of cooked foods versus raw foods on the immune system and performance. One study, conducted in 1930 under the direction of a Swiss medical doctor, Dr. Paul Kouchakoff, was reported in his paper entitled "The Influence of Food Cooking on the Blood

Formula of Man" and presented in Paris at the First International Congress of Microbiology. His findings showed that after a person eats cooked food, his or her blood responds immediately by increasing the number of white blood cells. This is a well-known phenomenon called "digestive leukocytosis," in which there is a rise in the number of leukocytes, or white blood cells, after eating. Since digestive leukocytosis was always observed after a meal, it was considered to be a normal physiological response to eating. No one knew why the number of white cells rises after eating, since this appeared to be a stress response as if the body was somehow reacting to something harmful, such as infection, exposure to toxic chemicals, or trauma.

Around the same time, Swiss researchers at the institute of Chemical Chemistry found that eating raw, unaltered food did not cause a reaction in the blood. In addition, they found that if a food had been heated beyond a certain temperature (unique to each food), or if the food was processed (through refinement or by adding chemicals, for instance), it always caused a rise in the number of white cells in the blood. The researchers renamed this reaction "pathological leukocytosis," since the body was reacting to highly altered food. They tested many different types of foods and found that if the foods were not refined or overheated, they caused no reaction. The body saw them as "friendly foods." However these same foods, if heated at too high a temperature, caused a negative reaction in the blood, a reaction found only when the body is invaded by a dangerous pathogen or trauma.

Professor Karl Eimer, director of the Medical Clinic at the University of Vienna, studied the effect of a 100% raw diet on athletes. He placed his subjects on a two-week program of intense physical training while they continued to consume their usual cooked diet. Their athletic performance was monitored and evaluated. They were then put on a 100% raw diet and continued their training. Without exception, the athletes demonstrated improvements in reflex speed, flexibility, and stamina. Eimer and his colleague Professor Hans Eppinger concluded that raw foods increase cellular respiration and efficiency. Their findings were reported in the July 1993 edition of *Zeitschrift fur Ernahrung* entitled "Klinik Schwenkenhacher."

When you are not getting the optimal nutrients out of your food, it becomes compromising. Even more so because vegetables are often cooked with oils, animal products, salt or sugars, making the effect even worse. If you do eat cooked veggies, keep it simple and lightly cooked, but it's better to try to eat the majority of your leafy greens and veggies raw

Q: You are a big proponent of orange juice as a part of the OTM plan, but to me you jokingly refer to "dead juice" as being juice that is not fresh squeezed. Why are citrus juices so good for us, and what's wrong with that fresh squeezed, not from concentrate juice we see in supermarkets.

A: Like cooked vegetables, juice from a bottle, can, or carton is unfortunately a compromising food. Why? Because the juice has probably gone through the process of oxidation. With oxidation, the juice changes chemical composition and loses its nutritional value, just like the changes that take place when vegetables are cooked. This is even more unfortunate, because citrus juices, especially orange juice, are great for your health.

Vitamin C from orange and other citrus juices is associated with a reduced risk of colon and other forms of cancer. Vitamin C helps prevent DNA mutations caused by free radical damage that can result in cancer, especially in areas of the body where cellular turnover is especially rapid, such as the digestive system. Preventing DNA mutations translates into preventing cancer. Vitamin C also prevents the free radical damage that triggers inflammation and inflammatory conditions, such as asthma, osteoarthritis, and rheumatoid arthritis.

Free radicals also oxidize cholesterol. Only after being oxidized does cholesterol stick to the artery walls. Since vitamin C can neutralize free radicals, it can help prevent the oxidation of cholesterol.

A 248-page report, "The Health Benefits of Citrus Fruits," released December 2003 by Australia's Commonwealth Scientific and Industrial Research Organisation (CSIRO), reviews 48 studies that show a diet high in citrus fruit provides a statistically significant protective effect against some types of cancer.

A recent draft report by the World Health Organization, "Diet, Nutrition and the Prevention of Chronic Disease," concludes that a diet featuring citrus fruits also offers protection against cardiovascular disease.

One large U.S. study reviewed in the CSIRO report showed that one extra serving of fruit and vegetables a day reduced the risk of stroke by 4%, and this increased by 5–6 times for citrus fruits, reaching a 19% reduction of risk for stroke from consuming one extra serving of citrus fruit a day.

The CSIRO report also includes evidence of positive effects associated with citrus consumption in studies for arthritis, asthma, Alzheimer's disease and cognitive impairment, Parkinson's disease, macular degeneration, diabetes, gallstones, multiple sclerosis, cholera, gingivitis, optimal lung function, cataracts, ulcerative colitis, and Crohn's disease.

Finally, the CSIRO report notes that as low-fat, nutrient-dense foods with a low glycemic index, citrus fruits are protective against obesity, a condition which increases the risk of heart disease, certain cancers, diabetes, high blood pressure, and stroke and adds to symptoms of other conditions like arthritis.

An orange a day might help keep ulcers away, according to a study published in the August 2003 issue of the *Journal of the American College of Nutrition*. In this study, researchers evaluated data from 6,746 adults enrolled in the Third National Health and Nutrition Examination Survey from 1988–1994. Study participants with the highest blood levels of vitamin C had a 25% lower incidence of infection with *Helicobacter pylori*, the bacterium responsible for causing peptic ulcers and in turn, an increased risk for stomach cancer. Researchers are uncertain whether *H. pylori* lowers blood levels of vitamin C or if high blood levels of vitamin C help protect against infection—either way, eating an orange or drinking a glass of orange juice each day might help prevent gastric ulcers. The lead researcher in this study, Dr. Joel A. Simon at the San Francisco VA Medical Center, urges people who have tested positive for *H. pylori* to increase their consumption of vitamin C-rich foods since this might help them combat H. pylori infection.

The findings, presented in the *Annals of the Rheumatic Diseases* showed that those who consumed the lowest amounts of vitamin C-rich foods were more than three times more likely to develop arthritis than those who consumed the highest amounts. New research published in the August 2005 issue of the *American Journal of Clinical Nutrition* adds to the evidence that enjoying a daily glass of freshly squeezed orange juice can significantly lower your risk of developing rheumatoid arthritis.

It is very clear that oranges and other citrus fruits are great for your health. Remember, it's whole oranges or freshly squeezed orange juice that gives you what you need to prevent disease, so reach for the oranges and either eat them or juice them and don't even think about juice from a bottle, can, or carton.

Q: Why is it an issue to mix fruits or fruits and vegetables in a meal? Why do I want to keep from mixing compromising foods with nutritious foods? Won't the nutritious foods just get absorbed into the body and do their good work?

A: It's not what you eat, it's what you digest and assimilate that counts. So, even when you eat life-enhancing food, you can combine them in such a way where they can be difficult to digest. The reason is that carbohydrates, fats, and sugars require different chemical processes for digestion. Sometimes mixing them can create digestive problems and a decrease in nutrient assimilation. There are definite combinations to avoid. I'll give you a few.

Complex carbohydrates (pasta, bread, rice, and potatoes) with acidic fruits (citrus and tomatoes).

The digestion of acidic fruits inhibits the digestion of complex carbohydrates and causes fermentation.

Complex protein with acidic fruits.

For the same reason as with complex carbohydrates, the digestion of the acidic fruits inhibits the digestions of the protein and causes fermentation.

Two or more concentrated proteins (fish, meat, nuts, or seeds).

All protein breaks down differently in the body.

Carbohydrates (complex, sweet fruits, and concentrated sugars) with concentrated protein.

Protein digestion can completely stop carbohydrate digestion because of the increased acidity in the stomach.

Concentrated fats (cream, butter, and oil) with concentrated protein.

Fat depresses the action of the gastric glands and inhibits these juices needed for protein digestion.

Milk.

Milk digests in the duodenum and should not be combined with anything else.

Melons.

Melons, due to their high water content and rapid breakdown, should be eaten alone.

Q: What about eating compromising foods? You mentioned eating them with a salad. That seems to contradict what you said about mixing foods. Why should we follow this approach?

A: On the OTM plan you will make choices about enhancing and compromising foods. The absolute healthiest choice is a meal of a single fresh, raw fruit or vegetable. Most of you will find that you will want to add some compromise in the form of cooked foods. Remember that cooking foods destroys most enzymes because the enzymes are proteins and sensitive to heat. When you eat compromising meals, especially those containing concentrated protein or complex carbohydrates, you will want to include a green salad. The greens will supply needed enzymes to help you with digestion. Eating a healthy green salad you're your compromising food or better yet, before the compromising food also helps you limit the quantity of compromising food you eat. So to get the most from your foods, don't mix them. But if you really want to eat that steak or a dish of pasta, remember to eat them with a big green salad.

Q: The OTM plan seems to incorporate the belief that the body has a tremendous power to keep itself healthy. It's a bit cliché, but maybe *an apple a day keeps the doctor away*, was more insightful than I imagined. Why do you think that this focus on nutrition and toxicity isn't a more widely held belief or more widely practiced?

A: We are focused on treatment, drugs, and supplements—anything that is outside our control. We are taught by Western medicine and food, drug, and supplement companies. They tell us that we need their products or services, and we believe them.

"Eating compromising foods has been shown to cause our bodies to deteriorate, yet eating fresh fruits and vegetables has never once been said to cause disease."

It is a question exactly how this belief got started - probably through effective and aggressive advertising. However, I do know that human beings and animals alike will do anything to avoid pain. We, as consumers, want to believe there is a cure, a product, or a magic treatment that we get us and keep us healthy. We want to be convinced that by taking a pill we will be disease and pain free. Some of these beliefs have been passed on to us for generations. We need to get the right information and let go of the beliefs that are not serving us.

Now, Western medicine is doing more research in the connection between disease, diet, and lifestyle and has passed that research to us, and our beliefs are slowly starting to change. When I look at this research, it makes me wonder why we wouldn't all change our beliefs immediately. Eating fried foods, animal products, concentrated sugars, and complex carbohydrates has been shown to cause our bodies to deteriorate, and yet eating fresh fruits and vegetables has never once been said to cause disease or accelerate aging. It's time to challenge the beliefs.

Here's an interesting story about hanging onto beliefs. I go to my eye doctor every 2–3 years for a checkup. My motivation to go is to check and see how much better my vision is getting. Every time I go in for my appointment, we have the same conversation:

Doctor: I don't understand how your eyes are getting better.

Me: I do my eye exercises, let my eyes get indirect sunshine, and use my glasses only when I absolutely need them.

Doctor: As I recall, we are the same age and I am impressed by your excellent close vision. That's not common at our age.

Me: I don't think my age has anything to do with my vision or yours. If you would stop wearing your glasses all the time and exercise your eyes, your vision would probably get better and you certainly wouldn't need bifocals. Why don't you try it just for a month?

Doctor: I just can't believe it would help.

We will have this conversation next year too! These questions are just a small example of the beliefs that keep us unhealthy and on a path to accelerated aging. You can change those beliefs and if you do, you will change your life.

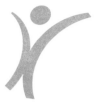

Stephen's OTM Food Checklist:

I was starting to see some ways I might be able to make the plan work for me and maybe for many of you as well. Here's how I was beginning to put it together:

- ✓ I have control over what I choose to eat and drink. I can make healthier choices.

- ✓ More healthy choices are better, and no healthy choices are the worst. I can find a level that works for me and still be better off than I am now.

- ✓ If I understand what nutritious food is right for me, I can make sure I get some at least every day in a way that I get maximum nutrition from that food. This should also help me be less prone to eating empty calories or compromising foods.

- ✓ If I understand what compromising food is, I can make choices on how to optimize my compromises and really enjoy them. I should choose great wine, the best chocolates, or a fantastic steak over cheap wine, candy bars from the vending machine, or a fast food burger.

- ✓ There are ways to eat compromising foods in smaller quantities and in combination with nutritious foods to minimize toxicity and still get all the enjoyment.

I think I see how the OTM plan can fit anybody's lifestyle. The idea is to choose a healthy target level. Say 50% OTM PLAN target. Make the choices necessary to ensure that 50% of the foods you eat are nutritious foods and are consumed in a way that allows them to make their full contribution to your health. Now what's needed is a framework to make it work.

OTM
Food Plan

How you incorporate the OTM plan into your life is important. It has to fit with your current lifestyle. If you want to change your lifestyle, you can take steps to do that. For now, though, you have to start exactly where you are.

The changes that you make have to feel good to you, or they won't become part of your life. For whatever reasons, you have to *want* to make these changes. You'll value things more if you do them for yourself because you want to do them. You have to feel satiated. If you feel deprived, the change won't last very long. If the food doesn't taste good to you or you don't incorporate the level of variety you need, it definitely won't last.

That's why I feel that diets are dead ends. This food plan is about increasing the amount of nutrients by adding life-enhancing foods to your meals in keeping with your personal lifestyle.

How the Framework Functions

Most people want to be healthy but are not ready, willing, or even interested in living on meals that consist of 100% fresh, raw, organic fruits and vegetables, 100% of the time. We all want to be healthy, yet we still enjoy those compromising goodies. We want our lives to be filled with possibilities, variety, and maybe a little decadence. This is exactly why we created this plan. The framework helps you find and maintain the levels that fit your lifestyle, and it also helps you progress toward our OTM plan goals for looking better, feeling great, and leading a happier and healthier life.

Here's how it works. The OTM plan is a tool to add more nutrients to your meals. Unlike diets, this plan is not about stopping yourself from enjoying what you love, but about helping you make healthy choices so that you can have energy to really enjoy your life.

For that reason, the OTM plan framework is focused on how much enhancing foods you add to your meals and how often you add them. It is a points-based framework that you can use on a daily or weekly basis to help you keep track of your nutritious meals. The structure is pretty simple. Each meal you eat in a day is worth 10 points and each snack is worth 5 points. Each day is worth a total of the aggregated points for the meals and snacks you have eaten.

For example, if you have breakfast, lunch, an afternoon snack, and dinner, then the total possible points would be 35, (10+10+5+10=35 points). If you have a 100% nutritious meal or snack for each one of these meals you would have 35 of 35 points for 100% OTM plan. If you have mostly enhancing meals or some enhancing and some not-so-enhancing, then you would have less than the 35 example points. Let's say you have 20 points out of 35 points. Then you are at nearly 60% OTM plan. If that is your chosen target, then you are right on plan!

The OTM plan framework is based on meals or snacks. What makes a meal nutritious or compromising is the proportion of nutritious to compromising foods. A meal of 100% nutritious foods is a 100% meal. For the purposes of the framework, at least 75% nutritious foods is the basis for earning some points. What you decide what to eat for the other 25% will determine the points you get. Fewer compromising foods will earn more points, while more compromising foods earn less or maybe none. It's okay though, because you might be able to balance that decadent meal with a couple of nutritious meals during the day.

When considering compromising foods for meal values, the framework separates these foods into two groups. Group A is less compromising and earns more points in combination with nutritious foods. It's the best choice when you are craving decadence.

Group B are foods that are much more difficult to digest and have the lowest nutritional values, but even these foods may make up part of your lifestyle if these are the compromises you choose, so they play a part in the OTM plan framework.

Compromising Food Group A (cfA)

- Cooked, but not fried, fruits and vegetables. Lightly steamed is better than boiled.
- Raw goat or sheep dairy (milk and cheese)
- Legume
- Rice
- Potatoes
- Raw nuts and seeds
- Dried fruits and veggies
- Olives

Compromising Food Group B (cfB)

- Beef, lamb, pork, etc.
- Poultry
- Seafood
- Cow dairy
- Pasteurized goat and sheep dairy
- Eggs
- Fried foods
- Wheat (bread, pasta, pizza, etc.)
- Roasted nuts and seeds

The OTM plan also considers that different people are coming to the plan with different lifestyles. For that reason, the plan has phases. Each phase is a bit more rigorous than the next, and each has a specific purpose. Some people will work their way through all phases, and some will find the phase that suits their lifestyle the best.

The OTM plan is all about increasing the nutrients in your body and cutting down toxicity and malnutrition. This is a plan about how much good stuff you can introduce into your life. At any phase and any level in the OTM plan, you are helping yourself to lose weight, look great, and lead a healthier and happier life.

Choosing Your Target Level

The OTM plan has three phases so that it can work for everyone. Each phase is designed for you to work with where you are, at your own pace and comfort level, so that you can comfortably introduce more nutritious and healthful foods into your life. Depending on your lifestyle, you might work your way from phase to phase, or you might find a phase that is most comfortable for you to live with. It's all up to you, because however you decide to adopt the plan, you will be better off than before.

Phase 1 is to help you make the transition. The objective of Phase 1 is to help introduce nutritious foods into your lifestyle and to help you choose nutritious foods over compromising foods.

In Phase 2 of the program most people could live without ever feeling deprived. The objective of Phase 2 is to increase the amount of nutrition in your diet and basically eat a higher percentage of nutritious foods than compromising foods.

Phase 3 might be your goal, or it might be a phase to try occasionally to increase your health and energy levels. The objective of Phase 3 is to live on enhancing foods most of the time with comprising foods on occasion.

Remember, the OTM plan is about winning. Even if you only add one life-enhancing meal a week, you have increased your nutrients by a certain percentage.

Also, whatever Phase you choose; try to drink an 8 ounce glass of distilled water before each meal to keep your body sufficiently hydrated.

Let's start with your current lifestyle:

In a week, how many times do you make a complete meal out of one of the following? (Don't include snacks.)

- Fruit
- Fresh-squeezed orange juice
- Raw vegetables
- Simple salads—mostly leafy greens without cheese, meat, or creamy dressings

If you answered:

0–2: Start at Phase 1

3–6: Start at Phase 2

6 and above: Phase 3

I'm going to take you through each winning phase; you can jump in anywhere you want.

Phase 1 – A Great Way to Start

I started out in Phase 1. Like some of you, the number of my enhancing meals was zero. The only fresh green vegetable on my plate was a parsley garnish and I threw that out before digging into my Philly cheesesteak dripping with hot oil.

Winning in Phase 1 is about adding nutritious foods into your meals and learning to make some trade-offs between nutritious and compromising foods. In the OTM plan framework, each meal you eat is worth 10 points and snacks are worth 5 points. The point system in Phase 1 is as follows:

- Award yourself 10 points plus a 5-point bonus if your meal consists of 100% enhancing food.

- Award yourself 10 points plus a 5-point bonus if your meal consists of at least 75% enhancing food, by volume, and no more than 25% from compromising food group A.

- Award yourself 10 points if your meal consists of at least 75% enhancing food, by volume, and no more than 25% from compromising food group B.

- Award yourself 5 points if you add one enhancing food—fresh, organic, raw fruits or vegetables—to any meal.

- Award yourself 5 points for each snack that consists only of enhancing foods.

- 0 points are awarded for any compromising snack.

Here's an example:

Say you eat 3 meals and 2 snacks.

Breakfast—Drinking 8 ounces of fresh-squeezed orange juice with your eggs and bacon and toast earns you 5 points.

Mid-morning snack—An apple for 5 points.

Lunch—A large green salad plus a baked potato, earns you 10 points plus 5 bonus points.

Dinner—Asmall salad, rice, a medium-sized steak, and grilled mushrooms is worth 5 points.

After-dinner snack—Chips and a beer for 0 points.

The total for this day is 30 points, (25 points plus a 5 point bonus), out of a possible 40 points. You would be at 75% Phase 1. Once you get to a level where you are consistently over 50% Phase 1, it might be time to move to Phase 2.

Phase 2—Balance That Can Change Your Life

In Phase 2, you are beginning to make determined trade-offs between nutritious and compromising foods. You are balancing nutritious meals with the compromising goodies you enjoy, and you might be incorporating some 100% enhancing meals or snacks into your lifestyle on a regular basis. Here's how Phase 2 works:

- Award yourself 10 points plus a 5 point bonus if your meal consists of 100% enhancing food.

- Award yourself 10 points if your meal consists of at least 75% enhancing food, by volume, and no more than 25% from compromising food group A.

- Award yourself 5 points if your meal consists of at least 75% enhancing food, by volume, and no more than 25% from compromising food group B.

- Award yourself 5 points for each snack that consists only of enhancing foods.

- 0 points are awarded for any compromising snack.

Here's an example:

Say you eat 3 meals and 2 snacks.

Breakfast—A 16-ounce glass of fresh-squeezed orange juice and a bowl of blueberries earns you 10 points plus a 5 point bonus,

Mid-morning snack—An apple for 5 points.

Lunch—Half of a turkey sandwich and a large salad, earning you 5 points.

Dinner—A small salad, baked potato, a medium-sized steak, and grilled mushrooms for 0 points.

After-dinner snack—An oh-so-decadent piece of chocolate and two glasses of wine over the rest of the evening earns you 0 points.

The total for this day is 25 points, (20 points plus a 5 point bonus), out of a possible 40 points. Your would be at 62.5% Phase 2. If you keep this up, you'll be ready for Phase 3!

Phase 3—You Are a Master Over the Myths

In Phase 3, you have comfortably managed to include nutritious foods into your life. You can and do include 100% enhancing meals and snacks into your day on a regular basis. You know your favorite compromises and enjoy them completely while keeping good nutrition as your guideline.

- Award yourself 10 points if your meals consist of 100% enhancing food.

- Award yourself 5 points if your meals consist of at least 75% enhancing food, by volume, and no more than 25% from compromising food group A.

- Award yourself 5 points for each snack that consists only of enhancing foods.

- 0 points are awarded for any compromising snack.

- 0 points are awarded for any foods from compromising food group B.

Here's an example:

Say you eat 3 meals and 2 snacks.

Breakfast—A 16-ounce glass of fresh-squeezed orange juice and a bowl of blueberries earns you 10 points.

Mid-morning snack—An apple for 5 points.

Lunch—A large salad with mango and avocado, earning 10 points.

Dinner—A large salad with raw sheep cheese for 5 points.

After-dinner snack—A small piece of flourless chocolate torte and a glass of wine over the rest of the evening earns you 0 points.

The total for this day is 30 points out of a possible 40. You would be at 75% Phase 3.

You can add more energy and nutrients to your body by substituting an enhancing meal for a compromising meal. The more enhancing meals you substitute, the better you will look and feel. By making just a few minor changes at any phase, you can increase your nutritional intake by 10–30%, which could translate to 10–30% healthier with that much more energy to enhance your life.

OTM Food Tip

The best choice for an enhancing food to add in combination with compromising food group A or B is a leafy green salad.

Point chart for all phases

	Phase 1	Phase 2	Phase 3
All enhancing foods (ef)	10 + 5 bonus	10 + 5 bonus	10
75% ef + 25% cfA	10 + 5 bonus	10	5
75% ef + 25% cfB	10	5	0
Adding ef to any cf	5	0	0

Point Chart Legend

ef= enhancing food
cf= compromising food
cfA= compromising food group A
cfB= compromising food group B

Stephen's Cheat Sheet for the OTM Food Plan:

Here are a few things that helped me adopt the OTM plan and stay with it:

✓ Breakfast seems to be the easiest meal to make all-enhancing and add good nutrients to our lives. Put off that cup of coffee until mid-morning and score yourself 10 points or more.

✓ Snacks are also a great way to add nutrients to a day. Have an apple or some other fruit during the day or when you get home at night. It adds points and you're likely to be less hungry when it comes to meal time.

✓ Cutting back on the salt makes a big difference. It's easy to replace with herbs and spices, and dropping it really helps you lose weight and keep hydrated.

✓ When eating any meal, have your nutritious foods first. Have a salad as an appetizer before digging into a nice grilled salmon filet. Remember to balance 75% salad to 25% compromising food – so you'll probably need to eat an entire garden to balance that 24 oz. porterhouse steak!

✓ Achieving 50% to 75% of any phase in the OTM plan is something to feel good about, and it's not that hard. A good breakfast, a decent snack, and at least one other five-point meal and you have made it for a typical day.

✓ When I look at a menu, I pick some taste that I want to make the special part of the meal and then I balance the rest. If it is an appetizer, then I have a salad entrée. If it's an entrée, start with a big mixed green salad with olive oil.

✓ If I know I am going to splurge at a meal—say during a special family dinner, or if I just want to treat myself to some decadence—I try to make my other meals and snacks that day count for high points. I can handle a zero point meal if I have already cleared my target for the day.

✓ Wine is a compromising food -so what! We all choose our compromises...

OTM
Meal Tips

I have never felt limited in my food choices on this plan. There is an amazing variety of fresh fruits and vegetables, and I can find great ingredients for a fantastic meal at any time of the year. Once you start on the plan, you will begin to taste and appreciate the difference fresh, natural foods can make. You might doubt it now, but just wait and see…you will love it!

Still, you are accustomed to eating another way, so as you start the OTM plan it might be helpful to have a few resources to draw upon to help you bring more nutrition into your life and the lives of those you love. An entire book could be dedicated to OTM-friendly recipes and foods, so maybe it will be the next book I'll write. Meanwhile, keep an eye out on the Web site (roegallo.com) for new recipes, tips, and techniques to help you to adopt the OTM plan.

STEPHEN ASKS:

Imagining meals that conform to the plan might take some getting used to. After all, I have a lifetime of habits around comprising foods. Thinking about the OTM plan as a way to add nutrition to my diet, are there any substitutes or things I can do with the preparation of what I eat that can help me?

The OTM Plan can be a gradual process. As you go through the phases, you will get used to eating more fresh fruits and vegetables, and the good news is you'll be washing fewer pots and pans! The little things can make a big difference in the OTM plan, so here are some ideas to transform a compromising meal into a less compromising or more enhancing one.

OTM Transform-a-Meal

Preparation and Serving Techniques

Before OTM	*The OTM Way*
Frying foods	Cooking foods reduces nutritional value, and frying foods is the most compromising. Consider grilling or baking instead of frying if you are going to cook something. The cooked oils in frying are one of the heaviest and least nutritious items you can eat. You can make a big difference just by cutting down fried foods.
Sandwiches	Use romaine lettuce, nori sheets, or corn tortillas to make wraps instead of sandwiches with bread. They're lighter and just as satisfying.
Chips for dipping	Try Romaine lettuce or Belgian endive for dipping instead of chips. I particularly love this with guacamole. Carrots, celery, and bell peppers work equally well.
Crackers for cheese	Sliced apples, pears, figs, and dates can be served with cheese instead of crackers. You get a both a great

complementary taste and better nutrition.

Candy and sweet snacks	Have a date roll instead of candy. Dates are wonderfully sweet, and there are several types of date rolls with great additions like coconut, pecans, and walnuts.

Substitution Items

Wheat flour	Substitute corn flour for wheat flour (for example, have corn tortillas instead of wheat tortillas)
Cow dairy	Use goat's milk or sheep and goat cheeses instead of cow's milk or cow cheese. Goat and sheep milk is much more easily digested, and the sheep and goat cheeses are delicious.
Sodas	Have a glass of fresh-squeezed orange juice, grapefruit juice, or homemade lemonade instead of soda.
Prepared salad dressing	Use pure extra-virgin olive oil instead of salad dressings. Virgin olive oils from around the world have wonderfully different flavors, so you'll not lack variety.
Vinegar	Try fresh-squeezed lemon instead of vinegar. It's great in salads and on vegetables.
Cooked tomatoes	Sun-dried tomatoes instead of cooked tomatoes make fabulous

sauces with great intense flavors. Try blending fresh and sundried tomatoes with virgin olive oil to lighten the sauce.

· Salt

Grind dried wakame seaweed in a small food processor and use it instead of salt. There are also prepared salt substitutes made from kelp that provide taste enhance ment at up to 10 times less sodium than normal table salt or sea salts.

Black pepper

Use cayenne pepper instead of black pepper. Black pepper is much more difficult to digest. Doing this, you get all of the pepper flavor—maybe even more intense—and you have a healthier source of spice.

Cream for sauces

Raw macada-mia or raw cashew nuts mixed in a food processor until you have a buttery consistency makes for a great thickener or cream sub-stitute for sauces or soups.

Sugar

Substitute agave nectar or honey to add sweetness to your drinks, dishes, and desserts.

Whipped cream

Blending banana with raw macada mia nuts and agave nectar makes a richly decadent and healthier alter native to whipped cream or dairy ice creams.

Ice cream	Consider sorbets as an alternative. They are compromising sugar foods, but you cut out the diary. I also recently found a non dairy ice cream made from coconut milk. It's fabulous! People in San Fran cisco can try Maggie Mudd at 930 Courtland Ave in San Francisco.

All the cooks among you have made terrific kitchens and know it makes a huge difference to have the right equipment. The same is true for preparing fantastic OTM plan dishes. Here are some of the items I have in my kitchen that make life much easier, and my dishes turn out terrifically.

Equipment:

Vita Mix blender

For most of these blended recipes you need a Vita Mix blender. If you're going to have a blender, it's the only one worth having. It's the only blender that actually blends everything, and it lasts forever. I've had mine for over 15 years and it's still going strong. If you don't have a Vita Mix, don't try the recipes that say Vita Mix because they won't blend properly and therefore won't taste the way they should.

Food processor

I like to have both a small and large food processor. They work great for sauces, nut butters, pesto, and much more.

Citrus juicer

You can spend anywhere from $15 to $200. I've been using the $15.00 model that holds up to 32 ounces, although I've been looking at a higher-end brand. I'll keep you posted on my Web site.

STEPHEN ASKS:

Roe, I can't eat another plain green salad. You must have some secrets about interesting salad combinations or other healthy dishes that I can eat that are more like the foods I was accustomed to eating. Tell me there is something beside a green salad in my future. Please!

Remember that the OTM Plan is a nourishment-focused plan, not a diet. You can eat anything you want. You just have to balance the amount of compromising food you eat with a healthy amount of nourishing food. So don't worry about making sacrifices. You will find that you won't feel you're making any sacrifices. I have found no shortage of variety in the types of salad combinations I can make, particularly if you add a little compromising goodie to the mix.

Still, as you move through the phases of the OTM plan you might want to make more trade-offs between nutritious foods and compromising foods. In that context, being creative with healthy, nutritious foods will be fun and can help balance the trade-offs. The great cooks among you will come up with wonderful combinations of fresh fruits, interesting salads, and dishes made with fresh vegetables. Experiment and remember to combine fruit with fruit and/or leafy greens (lettuces and herbs) and vegetables with vegetables and/or leafy greens. It's better not to combine fruit with vegetables other than leafy greens. Also, try to use nuts sparingly as they are a compromising food even when raw.

To help get you started here are some ways to add variety to your salads and some recipes I have found to be delicious and great ways to bring a creative and healthy flair to the OTM Plan.

If you have any OTM-friendly recipes that you believe to be fabulous, please send them to me with your name. If I choose one of your recipes for my website, I'll send you an OTM gift.

Salads

Salads along with fruits are the foundation foods of the OTM plan. Making salads interesting starts with your choice of leafy greens. There are a wide variety of lettuces and herbs that you can use in combination to create interesting and new taste sensations. Try the leafy greens combinations plain or mix them with fresh herbs for even more variety.

Garnish your salads with guacamole, corn salsa, tomato salsa, pesto or other fresh condiments. Add raw vegetables. Bring zesty flavor to a salad with a fresh lemon, orange, or lime splash. Try different olive oils; their flavors vary greatly from olive type, to region to time of harvest.

In addition, try some of these salad ideas:

Avocado Mango Salad

Ingredients

1 medium haas avocado

1 medium mango

Tips

This salad is great by itself or you can serve it over greens. I love it over arugula with a drizzle of fresh squeezed orange juice for a dressing. YUM!!!

Directions

Slice the avocado and mango into similar shapes. Depending on your preference for cubes or strips. Either mix the two fruits or place both on a plate and drizzle a little bit of fresh squeezed orange juice over the salad. Place over a bed or arugula lettuce to pair the sweet taste with the bitter leafy greens.

Avocado Cucumber Tomato Salad

1 medium avocado

1 medium tomato

1 small cucumber (skinned)

squeeze of fresh lemon or lime

Tips

To change the flavor sprinkle with a fresh herb (i.e. dill, chives, rosemary, parsley, cilantro, etc.).

Directions

Slice avocado into cubes and tomatoes and cucumbers into like-sized slices. Mix the ingredients together and squeeze fresh lemon over the salad. This also makes for a great addition to a plate of mixed leafy greens with a touch of olive oil.

. . . .

Tomato Basil Salad

Ingredients

4 ripe red tomatoes

fresh basil to taste

Tips

You can serve this salad by itself or over mixed greens.

Directions

Chop or finely slice tomatoes mix with basil and drizzle with olive oil.

. . . .

Dill Cucumber Salad

Ingredients

2 medium cucumbers

fresh dill to taste

squeeze of fresh lemon

Tips

You can serve this salad by itself or over mixed greens.

Directions

Chop or finely slice cucumbers, mix with dill and drizzle with olive oil and a splash of lemon juice.

. . . .

Mushroom Salad

Ingredients

12 ounces of mix fresh mushrooms

Parsley (Italian) to taste a small bunch

1 ½ ounce of sun dried tomatoes (reconstituted in hot water and pressed dry)

6 small tomatoes

1 clove of pressed fresh garlic

1 teaspoon of ground wakame

1 teaspoon of dried oregano

⅓ cup of olive oil

Tips

This salad stands on its own or can be served over lettuce. Change seasonings to create a completely different taste. Experiment.

Directions

Slice mushrooms, tomatoes, and sun dried tomatoes. Combine garlic, wakame, oregano and parsley with olive oil and mix.

. . . .

Sweet 'n' Succulent Kale and Avocado Salad

This is a great recipe from Karen Knowler. She made it for me when I was at her house in England. Check out her Web site at www.therawfoodcoach.com. Karen is amazing! The recipe is reprinted with the permission of Karen Knowler.

Ingredients

8 generous handfuls of green curly kale

Sprinkle of Celtic sea salt or Himalayan crystal salt

1–2 tablespoons of olive oil

1 ripe avocado

2 large tomatoes or a handful of cherry or baby plum tomatoes

OPTIONAL: 2 spring onions

OPTIONAL: 8 sun-dried tomatoes in oil

DRESSING: Squeeze of fresh lemon juice to taste

Tips

By adding the oil and salt to the leaves, the kale releases some of its moisture thereby making it much juicier in both taste and appearance. This treatment of kale makes it much more delicious and palatable, making all the difference for many people who ordinarily don't like kale as is.

Directions

Chop the kale into tiny pieces measuring roughly 1–2 cm square (approximately ½ -1 inch squares) and put into a bowl.

Add 1–2 tablespoons of olive oil plus a small sprinkling of your chosen salt to the kale and massage well into the leaves until they are glistening and look succulent. If they need more oil, add accordingly.

Chop one avocado into small pieces, add to the kale, and massage in well, coating the leaves. It is fine to leave pieces of avocado sitting amongst the leaves as well as coating them.

Chop tomatoes into small pieces and add to bowl. Similarly, finely slice the optional spring onions and sun-dried tomatoes—both of which I personally love.

Mix all ingredients well with your hands—a very tactile and delicious experience! Make sure that all ingredients are spread evenly throughout the bowl.

Sprinkle with some fresh lemon juice and serve as is or pile high on to a plate and garnish with tomatoes or olives.

Dressings and Dips

Corn Salsa

Ingredients

8 oz. of fresh raw corn

2 medium tomatoes (or 1/2 serving tomato salsa (see recipe)

1 medium avocado

fresh cilantro to taste

Tips

Raw corn is actually the fruit of the corn plant - cooking makes it difficult to digest.

This combination seems to digest easily.

If fresh corn is not in season, you can use frozen.

Directions

Place corn in a mixing bowl. Chop tomatoes and avocado and add to corn and mix. Add cilantro to taste.

• •

Guacamole

Ingredients

2 medium avocados

fresh tomato salsa to taste

Tips

Guacamole can be eaten as is, or:

• with a splash of fresh lemon or lime juice over lettuce

• stuffed into a hollowed tomato

• with raw veggies, celery or Belgium endive

• or as a filler for hearts of romaine.

Directions

Mash avocados, mix in salsa and serve.

Tomato Salsa

Ingredients

4 medium red tomatoes

½ small red chili

1 scallion (the green part)

cilantro to taste

squeeze of fresh lemon or lime

Tips

Increase or decrease the amount and type of peppers, depending on how "hot" you want it.

Directions

Chop tomatoes, chili and scallion. Squeeze in the lemon or lime and add cilantro to taste. Mix and serve.

. . . .

Tomato Sauce

Ingredients

1 cup Sun dried tomatoes

1 cup Fresh tomatoes

2 teaspoons of Olive oil

½ Red pepper

1 entire scallion

Basil to taste

Tips

You can make this sauce chunky or smooth and/or change the ratio of the ingredients, depending on the taste you want to achieve.

Directions

Chop sun dried tomatoes, fresh tomatoes, red peppers, scallion and basil in a food processor. Add olive oil and serve.

Pesto

1 ½ cup packed basil leaves

½ clove of garlic

¼ cup of pine nuts

¼ cup of pecorino cheese (to taste)

Approximately ¼ cup olive oil. (use enough to keep the mixture moist but not oily)

Tips

If you want a creamier pesto blend the garlic and pine nuts first until creamy then add basil, cheese and olive oil.

Try stuffing into hollowed mushrooms.

This recipe can be made without the cheese. Adding some lemon will balance the power of the basil.

Directions

Blend basil and garlic with a little olive oil until thoroughly chopped. Add nuts and cheese and blend again in the food processor.

. . . .

Cranberry Sauce

Ingredients

1 pound of fresh cranberries

⅓ cup of Agave (more or less to taste)

1 tablespoon of fresh mint

Tips

This can be served alone or over a bed of lettuce.

Directions

In the food processor chop cranberries and mint together using a pulsing action to leave coarsely chopped. Add agave to taste.

Avocado Mango Dressing or Avocado Mango Ginger Dressing

Ingredients

¼ avocado

1 mango

Optional: very small piece of ginger (to taste)

Tips

Add fresh squeezed orange juice if you prefer it thinner.

Directions

In a blender, blend 1/4 avocado, 1 mango (and ginger) until creamy.

· ·

Avocado Cucumber Tomato Dressing

Ingredients

1 avocado

1 cucumber

1 tomato

Splash of fresh lemon or lime juice

Herbs to taste

Tips

Add fresh squeezed orange juice if you prefer it thinner.

Directions

In a blender, blend all ingredients until creamy.

· ·

Tomato Basil Dressing

Ingredients

4 tomatoes

Basil to taste

Optional: Splash of fresh lemon

Tips

For a creamier dressing, add an avocado.

Directions

In a blender, lightly blend all ingredients. This is better chunky.

．．．．．．．．．．．．．．．．．．．．．．．．．．．．．．．

Dill Cucumber Dressing

Ingredients

2 Cucumbers (skinned)

Dill to taste

Optional: Splash of fresh lemon

Tips

For a creamier dressing, add an avocado.

Directions

In a blender, lightly blend all ingredients. This is better chunky.

．．．．．．．．．．．．．．．．．．．．．．．．．．．．．．．

Sun Dried Tomato Dressing

Ingredients

Sun dried tomatoes

Tomatoes

Herbs to taste

Optional: Splash of fresh lemon

Tips

For a creamier dressing, add an avocado.

Try with Basil, Dill, Cilantro, etc.

Directions

Soak sun dried tomatoes in hot water until soft. Pour off

water and blend in a food processor until smooth. Add chopped fresh tomatoes and fresh herbs and blend until creamy.

* *

Tomato and Basil Pesto

Take advantage of sweet, fresh tomatoes during the summer months to make this great dip for parties or as an appetizer before dinner. The tomato and basil combination is wonderful and the sun-dried tomatoes add a rich, intense flavor to the pesto. Serving the pesto on Belgian endive with a slice of avocado makes for a delicious first course. I also love this on my mixed green salads and topped with a bit of olive oil. Yum!

Ingredients

4 small red tomatoes

1 ounce of fresh basil

6 sun dried tomatoes

olive oil to taste

Tip (from the tomato snob)

Make sure tomatoes are sweet. Flavorless tomatoes are not worth eating. Also, never refrigerate fresh tomatoes. After the tomatoes have been made into a recipe, then you can store it in the refrigerator.

Directions

Reconstitute sun-dried tomatoes with hot (not boiling) water for about 30 minutes.

Blend all ingredients in food processor until tomatoes are chopped but still chunky.

Sushi

Avocado Maki

Ingredients

    1 cup Parsnips

    ⅓ cup Pine nuts

    3 Nori sheets

    1 Avocado

Tips

    Makes 3 rolls.

Directions

Wash and cut parsnips and put in food processor with pine nuts. Pulse   chop just until mixture looks like small pieces of rice. Do not over mix.

Peel an avocado and cut flesh into strips.

Place a nori sheet on your rolling mat and spread 1 cup of "rice" evenly over the nori by pressing with wet fingertips, leaving a 1 inch boarder at the top edge. Arrange several strips of avocado in the middle of the "rice"

Roll up the sushi tightly with the sushi mat to form a neatly packed cylinder (like a fat cigar)

Squeeze firmly to make sure the sushi roll is tightly packed.

Cut each sushi roll into 1 – 1 and ½ inch rounds using a sharp, damp knife. (moisten the knife in hot water after each cut)

Can be served with wasabi, soy sauce and/or ginger.

Fresh Soups

I'm including a recipe for corn soup, however, using the Vita-Mix Blender, you can put in just about any fruit or vegetable, add herbs and create delicious soups. You have no limits.

Fresh Corn Soup

During the summer months, you can take advantage of sweet fresh corn to make this simple and delicious soup. In the winter months, if you must have it, you can use frozen organic corn.

Ingredients (Serves 2)

> 6 ears of corn
>
> ¼ cup of water

Tips

Fresh corn should be sweet and juicy. If the corn has not been picked recently, it will be dry and not very flavorful—and so will the soup.

Directions

Shuck the corn, cut the kernels from the cob, add the water, and blend in the Vita Mix blender until it is warm.

Serve immediately and enjoy as is or top with fresh salsa and/or chopped avocado.

Shakes and Sweets

Breakfast Shake

Ingredients

> Any kind of fresh fruit in season
>
> Use ripe bananas for thickness.

Use distilled water, fresh coconut water and meat, or fresh squeezed orange juice.

Optional: organic dates

Do not mix more than three types of fruit.

If you peel and freeze the bananas in advance, your shake will come out even creamier.

Directions

Blend all ingredients in Vita Mix Blender just until smooth.

. . . .

Durian Pudding

Ingredients

Durian (can be fresh or frozen)

Tips

Pour into large wine glasses and serve slightly chilled. YUM!!!

Directions

Blend durian in food processor until smooth. (Don't over blend.)

. . . .

Stephanie's Date Balls

Ingredients

½ cup of raw nuts (macadamia, walnuts, etc.)

1 pound of dates

  rated coconut

Tips

Very decadent.

Great candy substitute.

Directions

Blend nuts in a food processor until soft but not buttery.

Add dates and blend until mixture forms a ball.

Make small balls and roll in grated coconut. Refrigerate.

. . . .

Banana Macadamia Cream

Ingredients

½ pound of raw macadamia nuts

4 frozen bananas

Tips

Use as a cream topping over fresh fruit (like blueberries).

Directions

Blend macadamia in food processor with regular blade until it turns into butter.

The nuts will go through a process of breaking up, balling up and finally breaking down to butter. Don't give up, it takes some time.

Break frozen bananas into small pieces and add slowly when still processing until all bananas are in and mixture is creamy.

. . . .

Raw and fabulous pie crust

Ingredients

1 cup of raw hazelnuts or macademia nuts

1 ounce of raw chocolate nibs

½ cup of dried coconut

3 ounces of Agave to taste

Tips

You can substitute the dried coconut for the raw chocolate. Use 1-cup total dried coconut for the entire recipe.

You can also eliminate the coconut completely.

Chop hazelnuts until fine

Add chocolate and pulse in food processor for a few seconds

Add Agave and process just until mixed

Press in 8 pie pan or individual dishes and refrigerate while making filling.

. . . .

Chocolate Mousse

Ingredients

½ cup Macadamia butter

1-2 bananas (depending if you like a banana taste)

½ cup of raw chocolate powder

3 ounces of Agave to taste

Tips

As a mousse: Fill wine glasses and chill.

As a filling: Fill piecrust and refrigerate.

Directions

Blend all ingredients together in food processor until smooth.

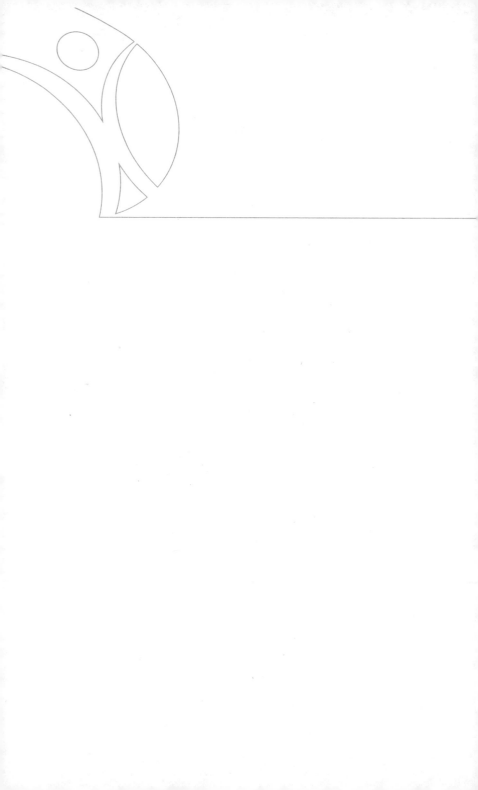

OTM
Exercise

The OTM plan must include exercise. In the chapter about the Flabby Myth, you learned that inactivity and not age was the issue. You can have a lean, fit, and flexible body and great muscle tone at any age—but you must exercise.

Exercise is physical movement for the purpose of making your body stronger and fitter. You have plenty of opportunity for exercise throughout the day. From the simplest of things like using the stairs instead of an elevator when possible, to taking a walk at lunch and taking small stretch breaks.

Physical movement also keeps you healthier, because it gives you energy by delivering more oxygen and nutrients to your cells. The positive effects of exercise are critical to defying the Sick Myth. You know the recommendations of the established medical community stating that physical exercise should be incorporated into plans for reducing the risk of heart disease, diabetes, cancer, stroke, and Alzheimer's disease.

Shortening the health span

A team of scientists at the USDA Human Nutrition Research Center on Aging at Tufts University. Dr. William Evans, chief of the Center's Human Physiology end Laboratory, and Dr. Irwin Rosenberg, director of the center, report that while inactivity doesn't necessarily shorten the life span, it most definitely shortens the health span.

According to the January 10, 2006, issue of *Annals of Internal Medicine*, recent studies reported that older people who exercised three or more times a week, including light aerobic exercise such as walking for 15 minutes, showed a lower risk of developing Alzheimer's and other types of dementia. One theory is that exercise might improve vascular function in the brain and/or reduce levels of amyloid, a sticky protein that clogs the brain in Alzheimer's patients. So now you need to make sure you are getting the beneficial exercise you need.

"The less physically active people become as they advance in years, the faster their bodies give out on them."

Start by finding things you love to do and then doing them. The key here is enjoying what you do. Exercise is supposed to be fun, so don't make it a chore. Playing sports, dancing, climbing, swimming, and running with your dog are just a few examples of fun exercises. Discover what fun is for you—what makes your body feel great.

In the OTM Fitness plan below, you will read about aerobic exercise and resistance training. These are only examples, so take note of the core concepts and tips and apply them to your favorite forms of exercise.

The OTM Fitness Plan

Along with the food plan, there are three stages of the fitness plan.

During Phase 1: Aim for at least 30 minutes of aerobic exercise once a week and 15 minutes of dedicated resistance training with or without weights.

During Phase 2: Aim for at least 30 minutes of aerobic exercise twice a week and two 15-minute sessions of dedicated resistance training with or without weights.

During Phase 3: Aim for at least 30 minutes of aerobic exercise three times a week and three 15-minute sessions of dedicated resistance training with or without weights.

Each of the exercise phases should include a warm-up and cool-down regimen.

Three Keys for Successful Exercising

Exercise should be fun, beneficial, and safe. Here are three simple but essential things to do to make the most of your exercise program and protect your body from injury.

The three key components for successful exercising are posture, flexibility, and conditioning.

Building a Strong Foundation

Building a strong body is like building a house—you have to start with the foundation. The foundation of your body is made up of your bones (especially your backbone), and your muscles. Your bones and muscles work together so that you can stand, sit, and move.

It is important to keep your body in alignment with good posture at all times and is crucial during exercise. Just like with a house, you have to make sure your foundation is straight and sturdy.

A strong, straight foundation will help keep your back healthy, your muscles relaxed, and your body free from injury. Also, great posture is the key for maintaining your height as you age.

STEPHEN ASKS:

I think I get the concept, but it's hard for me to know exactly what you mean. How about some tips for a strong foundation?

Here are some great tips for building and keeping a strong foundation.

Keep your pelvis in a neutral position with your lower abs and lower back muscles relaxed while sitting, standing, lying down, and walking. Pelvis in neutral position means that your pelvis is neither tipped too far forward nor too far backward. Also, unless the exercise naturally engages your lower abs or lower back muscles, you should maintain this position during exercise.

"Keep your feet pointed straight ahead."

Keep your feet pointed straight ahead when walking or running. This is important because when your feet are turned out, the hip flexor muscles are contracted, and a constant contraction of these muscles will ultimately lead to severe back problems. Keeping the hip flexors relaxed will keep your shoulders and hips aligned.

Keep your shoulders lifted up and back. If you contract your upper abs, you will stretch the middle back and your shoulders will drop. If you contract the middle back, it will pull your shoulders too far back.

Keep your spine in a straight line. If one of your oblique muscles—the muscles on the sides of your waist—is contracted, it will pull your spine out of alignment.

Keep your neck muscles relaxed. Play around with this one also. Move your head and see where you feel contractions in your neck muscles. Keeping the neck relaxed will keep it in alignment.

STEPHEN ASKS:

Trainers and sports magazines always talk about stretching. Is it really that necessary? I mean, I'm not doing triathlons here. Plus I find it takes up the time I have for exercising!

Flexibility is the second key component for successful exercising. Stretching is what keeps your body flexible. Think about why you exercise. You exercise because you want to improve your body, not harm it. If you work your muscles without stretching them first, you are putting yourself at risk for injury and if you are injured, there goes your exercise program.

Your muscles must be flexible so that they can move your bones on demand, and strong so that they can support your bones in any activity you care to participate in.

You need to be sufficiently aware of your body to recognize when your muscles need to move. When babies or animals—especially cats—wake up, the first thing they do is move their bodies very slowly. They wiggle and squirm, they yawn and make faces, and then they stretch. They're great to watch, and magnificent teachers as well. A yoga instructor once told me that the best yoga teachers were cats.

When you awake, your muscles need that same kind of gentle attention. Five minutes of movement and stretching can get the blood circulating and the muscles ready to start the day. Again, it's good to start out with slow, easy stretches and then move into holding a stretch. Always contract a tight muscle before stretching it!

Stretching lengthens your muscles and makes them more flexible. To keep your muscles flexible throughout your busy days, you need to periodically move and stretch them. Tight muscles pull your bones out of alignment, resulting in neck and back problems. Imagine being a cat and stretching every muscle of the body continually throughout the day.

There are a couple of types of stretching, and both types should be part of your OTM exercise plan. Dynamic stretches are slow, easy, continuous movements that stretch the muscles. Start your program with dynamic stretches because they gently wake up the muscles and slowly ease the muscles into a lengthening position.

Static stretches are stretches that are held. Here, the muscle is stretched then held in a lengthened position. Do static stretching during and after a workout to keep warm muscles lengthened.

Nice and Easy Does It

Conditioning your body means following a gradual training program to build strength and aerobic capacity. Conditioning is the third key component for successful exercising. It is important to start where you are and condition slowly; this way you will have a better opportunity to reach your fitness goals while staying injury free.

Six Weeks to Step-by-Step Aerobic Conditioning

Here's an example: If you want to start a running program and you can only run a city block, – that's great. Start with a goal of 20 minutes.

This six-week conditioning program can also work for other aerobic activities, like walking, dance, biking and other sports. Just substitute your favorite activity into this program.

Week 1

Walk for 5 minutes to warm up.

Walk for 20 minutes, each day increasing your speed until you can walk quickly (not running or jogging) for 20 min utes effortlessly. This might take more or less then a week to get there. Be patient.

Walk for 5 more minutes to cool down.

Week 2

Walk for 5 minutes to warm up.

Walk quickly (not running or jogging) for 20 minutes effortlessly.

Walk for 5 minutes to cool down.

Week 3

Walk for 5 minutes to warm up.

Walk quickly (not running or jogging) for 15 minutes effortlessly.

Run for 5 minutes.

Walk for 5 minutes to cool down.

Week 4

Walk for 5 minutes to warm up.

Walk quickly (not running or jogging) for 10 minutes effortlessly.

Run for 10 minutes.

Walk for 5 minutes to cool down.

Week 5

Walk for 5 minutes to warm up.

Walk quickly (not running or jogging) for 5 minutes effortlessly.

Run for 15 minutes.

Walk for 5 minutes to cool down.

Week 6

Walk for 5 minutes to warm up.

Run for 20 minutes.

Walk for 5 minutes to cool down.

If you feel you need more than one week before increasing the time you run, then take it. Do each step until it feels easy. Keep increasing slowing until you are running for 20 minutes. The key is to build up slowly and condition not only your muscles but your cardio-respiratory system as well.

Tip for aerobic workouts

What does effortlessly mean? It means that your inhale matches your exhale. You should be able to carry on a conversation during an aerobic workout.

Train Muscles From Large to Small

Muscles tire when they can no longer maintain a contraction. The larger muscles will last longer than the smaller ones. Therefore, you need to work large muscle groups first. For example, in resistance training you would start with the legs and back muscles, going on to the chest, shoulders, and then arms. In aerobic dance, the legs are worked before the arms. The intensity and duration of muscular contraction also plays a part in muscle fatigue. With regular resistance training, it is possible to do many more contractions than with power lifting, in which the intensity is much greater and the duration of a single contraction is much longer.

Make Time for Rest and Recovery

Rest is so important. You must make sure there are rest days built into your training program, no matter what level you are in the process. This is extremely critical when you are just starting a program or training hard. Muscles must recover or else temporary damage can set you back in our training and permanent damage will stop you permanently.

4 Steps to Stay Injury Free

1. Warm up before and cool down after exercising
2. Keep body in alignment during exercise
3. Condition heart and muscles
4. Rest and allow muscles to recover

If you do get an injury, you must rest and wait until you are healed before you proceed with a slow gradual training program until you are up to speed.

If your injury involves swelling, remember RICE—Rest, Ice, Compression, and Elevation.

You Don't Need a Gym

You have a built-in "body gym." Here is a great 55-minute workout that can be done at home or on the road.

The Great 55-Minute Workout

This workout covers everything. It's easy. It's fast. And it's thorough.

- Dynamic stretching: 5 minutes
- Warm-up: 5 minutes
- Aerobic activity: 20 minutes
- Cool down: 5 minutes
- Resistance training: 15 minutes
- Static stretching: 5 minutes

Stretching

Start with dynamic stretching. This should be the first part of your warm-up. Save the static stretches until you cool down.

Warm-Up

It is important to build up to an intense workout by slowly increasing the amount of blood being pumped to your cells. During strenuous exercise the blood flow to your muscles can increase to over 80 percent. The additional blood actually makes the muscles warmer and more flexible and gives them a steady increase in oxygen.

Examples of warm-up activities are walking, dynamic stretching, slow biking, and easy movement exercises.

Isotonics for Body, Face, and Eyes

Isotonics can be defined as the use of equal resistance throughout a range of movement. Push-ups, pull-ups, and weight-bearing exercises (free or fixed resistance) are all examples of isotonic exercise. I highly recommend isotonics, especially when you use your own body weight for resistance. A program of push-ups, pull-ups, squats, lunges, calf raises, abdominal crunches, and pelvic tilts—all done without weights—can be incorporated into your lifestyle. No gym is required. Also, isotonic exercises can be used to strengthen the face and eyes. Facial exercise will improve muscle tone and appearance. Contracting and relaxing the eyes strengthens your eye muscles and improves your vision.

Push-Ups

You can do full push-ups or push-ups with bent knees. Lay stomach down on the ground with neck, back, and buttocks in a straight line. Place hands under shoulders and lift body keeping neck, back and buttocks in a straight line. Using your stomach muscles will help you keep the proper form. Do in proper form until fatigued.

Crunches

Lay on your back with knees raised in the air and bent as if your legs were forming a step or placed upon the seat of a chair, but do not use a chair. Keep your eyes focused toward ceiling with your neck and back in straight line. Place your hands behind your head and raise your upper body a few inches until you feel your upper abdominal muscles contract. Do not pull up your head with your arms, the source of movement should come from upper abdominal contractions.

Pelvic Tilt

It is important that you practice the pelvic tilt as much as possible. Lay down with your knees bent and feet flat on the floor, or you can raise the buttocks off the floor to form what is called a bridge position. Rock the pelvis back toward your upper body by contracting the lower abdominal muscles. Do not use your back to raise the pelvis up. Think rocking. Repeat the rocking motion slowly until fatigued. The pelvic tilt is the best exercise for tightening the lower abs, toning the buttocks, and strengthening the lower back.

Lunges

While standing, place feet shoulder width apart and hands on waist. Step forward with one foot.

Slowly bend your other knee towards the floor, stopping just before touching the ground. Slowly return to your initial position by using your thigh muscles to lift yourself and straighten the bent knee. Having returned to the standing position, repeat the process starting with the other foot. Contract the abdominal muscles to help lift you and maintain balance. Lunges can be held as a stretch or done in a series until fatigued.

Squats

Start with the same position as used for lunges. Slowly squat down maintaining balance with a straight back and contracted abdominal muscles. Do not go beyond a 90 degree bend in the knees. Lower and lift yourself using muscles in your thighs and buttocks. Slowly return to standing and repeat until fatigued.

Isometrics

Isometric exercises are done with resistance but without movement. The key to isometrics is holding and intensifying the contraction without holding the breath. In isometrics you actually trick your brain into believing that you are doing work. In fact, whether you are pulling on or pushing against a mobile object or something stationary, your muscles work just as hard.

Doing isometric exercises while in bumper-to-bumper traffic is a great way to tone up the body while relieving stress. You can work on your abs or glutes or use the steering wheel for resistance to work on your arms and chest. Developing this habit takes some persistence. You can remind yourself by sticking a note on the car dashboard. Also, when you focus on isometrics rather than the traffic jam, you can get to your destination in better shape and stress-free.

Cool-Down

The cool-down will gradually slow the pumping action of your heart. Remember that during exercise, additional blood is being pumped to the muscles. You want this excess blood to be returned to our heart – gradually. If we stop exercising abruptly, blood may pool in the veins – causing pain and cramping. Examples of cool-down activities: Walking and stretching after heavy aerobic exercise (biking, running, etc.); and stretching after resistance exercises.

Care for the Eyes

The eye muscles are crucial for good vision. If your eye muscles are tight, you will not see distances well, leaving you nearsighted. If your eye muscles are overly relaxed, you won't be able to see well up close, leaving you farsighted. Vision therapy relaxes and strengthens the eye muscles. Corrective glasses and contact lenses are a crutch. They help you see better temporarily, but do not correct your vision. Vision therapy does work, even if someone is considered legally blind. Aldous Huxley and Meir Schnieder are perfect examples. These two high-profile men went from being legally blind to being able to see by practicing vision therapy.

I wore contacts because of my myopia (nearsightedness) and for severe astigmatism (irregularity of the surface of the eye). I could see fine close up, but three feet or further away from my nose, everything blurred. I also had terrible night vision. After reading Aldous Huxley's book *The Art of Seeing*, I threw out my contacts and immediately started the program that included sunning my eyes, palming, and blinking.

Instead of using my contact lens as a crutch, I started using my eye muscles. The first few months were challenging. I got a pair of regular glasses and wore them when I was driving or if I really had to see something. My vision gradually started to improve. I also read Dr. Bates' book, *The Bates Method for Better Eyesight Without Glasses*, as well as Meir Schneider's personal story. Schneider, who has a clinic in San Francisco, kept his legal-blindness certificate and likes to display it side-by-side with his driver's license.

I also highly recommend Tom Quackenbush's book, *Relearning to See*. Tom's book is the most comprehensive book ever written on the Bates method. If you want a thorough and practical self-help book on improving your eyesight, this is a great book to buy. Tom also teaches classes in the San Francisco area.

Poor vision habits take time to let go of, so be patient. Good vision is worth striving for. I can now see the leaves on trees from a distance without corrective lenses. In the sunlight, my vision is 20/20. At night I occasionally lose some clarity, especially if my eyes are tired. My vision is not perfect yet, after over 20 years, but it is so much better than it was and it keeps on improving and that's what important.

4 Steps to Great Vision

1. Sunning
2. Palming
3. Movement
4. Relaxation

Sunning

Sunning is done through lightly closed eyelids. Tilt your head toward the sun and rotate it left and right. This allows the sunlight to gently bathe the retina.

Palming

To palm, cup your hands over your closed eyes and visualize black.

Movement

I have a tendency to stare (the myopic stare), which causes the muscles of my eyes to stay contracted, hence the nearsightedness. Blinking, shifting, and moving help bring objects into focus by relaxing the eye muscles.

- Blink your eyes consciously—feel the opening and closing.
- Shift your focus from one object to another.
- Move your eyes over all parts of an object without focusing on the entire object at once.

Relaxation

- Rest in darkness. Soft, padded eye masks are great.
- Relax in general.
- Breathe.

Sunglasses

Sunglasses are particularly detrimental, as your body's ability to protect itself from excessive sun is linked to its natural perception of the sun's brightness. When it is sunny the pupil of the eyes contract, so the light is let in through a smaller opening. In the back of the pupil are melanin cells. When the sun's rays contact the pupils, the brain sends a signal to the melanin cells to release dark pigment throughout the entire body to protect the skin from sun damage. When you wear sunglasses, the dark lenses fool your eyes, interfering with your natural skin protection. Burning and skin cancer are the result. Use sunglasses only in dangerously intense glare situations, such as snow skiing and driving your car into the sun.

Facial Exercises

Laugh if you want, but I do them all the time—when driving in my car, while I'm brushing my teeth, and the list goes on. Your facial muscles are just as important as the rest of your muscles and need to be exercised. Facial exercises keep your facial muscles toned, providing adequate blood flow to your skin. If your muscles are not toned, your skin will eventually sag. Doing facial exercises will help keep your face looking healthy and alive. There are all types of facial exercises and even books on the subject. Watch children make faces or watch a man shaving. Use those muscles. It's a facelift without the stress and expense of surgery.

And, remember, a big part of looking great is healthy skin. People spend billions each year on skin care products and dermatology, especially for the face. They overlook the most important aspect of looking vibrantly healthy – good hydration. Keeping the water content of your cells high will keep your body healthier and reflect nicely on your skin. Cutting back on salt and alcohol and adding a glass of distilled water before each meal is better than a tube of skin cream anytime.

Brain Fitness

The brain needs nutrients and exercise just like the muscles in our body. Nutrients and exercise keep the brain healthy.

The most recent research on genetic predispositions to disease, including Alzheimer's, states that eating a healthy diet and exercising regularly are the best preventative actions you can take.

Using your brain will help will help it keep fit. Learning something new, reading, analyzing, and doing brainteaser puzzles, just to name a few, are some of the activities you can do to keep your brain fit.

Also, according to research in brain science today, especially in the area of psychoneuroimmunology, emphasis is being placed on how the mind—what you think and believe— considerably influences the health of your brain and, in turn, your entire body. If you believe you will always be mentally fit, you will naturally take the proper steps for keeping your brain and mind healthy because you move in the direction thoughts take you. Who you believe you are is who you become.

OTM
Mind

If you decide that you don't want to buy into the myths of aging, you must have the beliefs to support that decision. By the way, having made the decision means you are already well on your way to beating the myth of aging.

In the previous chapters, you learned how to be slim, fit, and healthy and how to feel sexy. Now in order to really make use of that information, you must believe it.

Your beliefs about aging determine your:

• attitude and the way you see yourself.

• emotions and how you feel about yourself.

• behaviors and the way you act out your life in your world.

• and, as a direct consequence of these actions, your results and the type of life you live.

Where Do Beliefs About Aging Come From?

Beliefs, in general, are based on information that comes into your mind. Outside sources, such as family, friends, religion, society, medical associations, science, education, and the media, can contribute to your beliefs. Most of your beliefs were formed when you were very young—much too young to be able to discern whether the beliefs were healthy, destructive, or even real.

Over the years, those beliefs are shaped or reinforced by your social and cultural environment. Today, most beliefs about aging are also influenced by marketing and advertising programs whose sole purpose is to sell products, services, movies, music, and drugs.

The good news is that you don't have to buy into a framework of beliefs that promote the aging myths. You can get the correct information, change your beliefs, and go on to really live a happier, healthier, and more powerful life.

The Beliefs Exercise

Here's a great exercise to begin to transform negative disempowering beliefs about aging, or any other negative belief, to more accurate, more positive, and much more empowering beliefs.

1. Make a list of all your beliefs about aging, positive and negative.
   - aging in general
   - aging and health
   - aging and weight
   - aging and fitness
   - aging and the ability to learn, change, and/or do
   - aging and sex

Next to the belief, write down where the belief originated (if you know).

2. Now review your list and ask yourself:
   - Does this belief empower me?
   - Does it really represent who I am and what I want?

If you answered "no" to any of the questions, you can write a powerful belief to replace the old disempowering belief. The new beliefs must be drilled into you just as the old beliefs were. You need to say your new beliefs over and over again to plant them firmly into your mind.

Here's an example. Say you have this belief:

Older people are frail. I'm going to have to have someone take care of me because I will be too weak to care for myself.

This belief is definitely not empowering and does not represent who you are or what you ultimately want for yourself. Plus it does not have to be true. You can change this belief to a more empowering belief and start taking the action steps to make it accurate:

I take great care of my body. I eat enhancing and nutritious foods, I exercise regularly and I maintain a great attitude about aging and about life in general. I'm smart about my aging and feel confident in my ability to take care of myself. I might actually be in better shape now than I was a couple of years ago.

Here are five steps that I found extremely helpful to empower my mind and therefore my life.

Five Steps to a New Attitude About Aging

1. Establish core beliefs
2. Practice positive self-talk
3. Choose to live on purpose
4. Laugh
5. Anticipate greatness

Step 1: Establish Core Beliefs

Your core beliefs are the foundation of all your other beliefs. Your core beliefs determine, among other things, how you live your life, how happy you are, and what type of relationships you have. By doing the beliefs exercise above, you can establish empowering core beliefs that can dramatically change your life.

Here are some of my personal core beliefs that keep me feeling young and powerful:

- Every day I'm alive is a great day.
- My life is filled with infinite love, health and energy.
- I have financial freedom and unlimited power.
- Everything that happens benefits me.
- The older I get, the better I get

Living with these core beliefs makes me happy to be alive. When I get stressed or angry, I can bring myself back to joy and gratitude by focusing on my beliefs. These beliefs keep me on track to take great care of myself.

If you do nothing else but this step, your life would change dramatically.

Step 2: Practice Positive Self-Talk

Self-talk is that little voice that speaks persistently and can sometimes be very negative. Communication with yourself must be positive, honest, loving, and respectful in order for you to be happy, healthy, and powerful.

Do you know your little voice? Does it sometimes get out of hand and say mean and nasty things to you? You must take control of your little voice because what you consistently say to yourself can reinforce or change your beliefs, create your life, and determine what you become. What you say, and what you see, is what you get.

Your little voice is on all the time, but do you pay attention to what it says? Do you think, "I'm getting old" or "I'm getting better at living"? Do you tell yourself, "I'm staying strong" or "I'm falling apart"?

You move in the direction of your most current and dominant thoughts.

Do you think, "I'm in control of my life" or "I'll never be able to do it, I'm too old"? If you tell yourself something is too hard, then it will be too hard, and you will not be able to achieve it. If you say you're too old, you will be—period!

Also, asking yourself empowering questions helps you find a great answer in every situation.

When you think about getting older, such questions as, "Why am I getting old?" drag you down so that you approach life from the standpoint of being helpless or being a victim. On the other hand, if you ask, "How can I make the most of my life?" or "What can I do to make myself better?" or "What are the benefits of aging?" you create a positive and powerful answer and outcome.

Step 3: Choose to Live on Purpose

To live on purpose means to live your life with passion and intention. It means that you don't put your life on hold. You take control and not let yourself be stopped by the myths of aging. To live on purpose means to make the most of every minute of every day.

Here are some great guidelines so that each day you can choose to live your life on purpose:

- Instead of letting fear paralyze me, I choose to let fear be my motivation for diving into life.

- Instead of waiting for things to happen, making excuses, or being a victim, I choose to take responsibility and make things happen. I choose to visualize what I want, set goals (especially daily goals), and take action.

- Instead of abusing myself or others or letting anyone abuse me, I choose to be positive, kind, gentle, loving, supportive, and respectful to myself and others and choose relation ships with people who are like-minded and love, support, and respect me.

- Instead of looking for what is bad or wrong, I choose to be grateful and to look for the good in everything that comes to me.

- Instead of buying into the myths of aging and letting my body and mind fall apart, I choose to take exceptional care of myself and live my life happier, healthier, and much more powerful.

Step 4: Laugh

Laughter is said to be the best medicine. Laughter keeps you young, healthy, positive, and loving. Laughter connects you with what is real, eliminates stress, and helps us not to take life so seriously.

Step 5: Anticipate Greatness

As you age, it is important to anticipate that you will add more greatness to your family, our friends, and the world in general.

Your life is significant and powerful, and you have a considerable influence on the quality of life around you. Greatness is not confined to winning the Nobel Peace Prize or saving millions from disaster. You can add greatness to the world in many ways.

You can change someone's life with a smile, a random act of kindness, forgiveness, and love. You can foster a loving and rich family life, mentor and lead in the workplace, create caring and joyful friendships, and give back to the community.

By living your life with intention to be great and to be the best you can be, each day can be a day to add a little more greatness to the world, just because you are alive.

YOU
and the World Around You

Your body is a temple of life. It is your greatest gift. It houses your life force - your connection to spirit, to others, to all of life. The more grateful you are for this incredible gift, the more you will respect, love and care for yourself, and the more joy you will have in your life. In following the OTM plan you demonstrate your gratitude for your body and who you are, and in doing so, reinforce your own ability to believe that you can have a wonderful life. By creating a healthy body you also create a healthier spirit. You witness how mind and body are connected, and see that it is not too late for you to have what you want in life. You also reinforce your connection to the world around you, and this in turn, will affect your compassion, respect and love for others, for nature and for our planet.

Imagine yourself in a beautiful garden. The trees are laden with luscious apricots, plums and peaches — all the fruits you love. The sun is shining and the day is balmy. A stream of fresh, clean water flows nearby. You quench your thirst. After taking a swim in the cool, refreshing water, you're hungry. Do you reach for the succulent fruit, or do you long for something packaged, processed, and artificial?

We now live in a way that is so detached from nature that we are completely unaware of what strange creatures we have become. By not taking care of our own body, we are not only in the process of destroying ourselves; we are also in the process of destroying our planet.

Just like our life support systems, the earths' life support systems are intertwined and their balance is necessary for the health of the entire planet and all creatures living on the planet. As we keep our internal environment free of toxins and waste to ensure our health, so too we need to consider keeping the earth – our external environment – free from toxins and waste as well.

One way we can do this is by paying attention to the way we eat. Here's why . . .

The food industry and the packaged, processed and canned foods that are produced add more waste and pollution. Cattle ranching is a major cause of deforestation, setting off a vicious cycle throughout the planet that contributes to global warming and that negatively affects our air quality and our water supply. Commercial agriculture drains and pollutes precious water and topsoil and uses a considerable amount of fossil fuel energy.

A 2002 study from the John Hopkins Bloomberg School of Public Health estimated that, using our current system of food production, an average of three calories of energy were needed to create one calorie of edible food. Grain-fed beef requires thirty-five calories for every calorie of beef produced. The study did not include the energy used in processing and transporting food, which could make the average jump to seven to ten calories of energy to produce one calorie of food.

"Sustainable farming can dramatically reduce fossil fuel consumption and pollution."

Energy is used for inefficient growing practices, food processing, and storage, as well as our system of transporting foodstuffs thousands of miles between the field and the end consumer. However, the biggest culprit of fossil fuel usage in industrial farming is the production of chemicals. In 2000, Martin Heller and Gregory Keoleian from the Center for Sustainable System at the University of Michigan, found that as much as forty percent of energy used in the food supply chain goes towards the production of artificial fertilizers and pesticides. To produce and distribute these chemicals takes an average of 5.5 gallons of fossil fuels per acre.

The United States Department of Agriculture estimates that making all our farmland's irrigation systems just ten percent more efficient would annually save eighty million gallons of diesel gasoline spent on pumping and applying the water. Also, reducing repetitive fertilizer application on the 250 million acres of major cropland in the United States would save approximately one billion dollars worth of petroleum-based fertilizers and pesticides. This practice would also prevent additional soil and water pollution.

According to the United States Department of Agriculture, we can achieve dramatic reductions in fossil fuel consumption and pollution through sustainable farming practices. Sustainable farming practices, sustainable agriculture, is defined by the University of California Sustainable Research and Education Department as follows:

Sustainable agriculture integrates three main goals--environmental health, economic profitability, and social and economic equity. These farming practices rest of the principle that we must meet the needs of the present without compromising the ability of future generations to meet their own needs. Therefore, stewardship of both natural and human resources is of prime importance. Stewardship of human resources includes consideration of social responsibilities such as working and living conditions of laborers, the needs of rural communities, and consumer health and safety both in the present and the future. Stewardship of land and natural resources involves maintaining or enhancing this vital resource base for the long term.

Supporting local and organic sustainable farmers and reducing the use of animal products and processed foods can benefit the planet and us, as well. Following these tenants of the OTM plan, the small changes we make as individuals are magnified as a group, and can make a meaningful contribution to the health of our planet and to life on earth.

FINAL
Words

You can have a healthy, fit, and active mind and body at any age by following the OTM plan and replacing disempowering beliefs and habits with healthy, powerful beliefs and habits.

You are never too old to be interesting, sexy, and stylish. You can always be up on what's new and what's happening in the news, music, art, and fashion. In fact, these are some of the things that keep you ageless and incredibly fascinating.

When you celebrate who you are and when you are spontaneous, flexible, and open to what life brings you, you defy the myths of aging by charting your own course in life.

Remember, you are never too old to do almost anything in life, especially when it comes to taking care of your body; changing old patterns; enhancing your mind; learning new things; and bringing greatness, joy, and love to your world. Acting now to change your diet will make all the difference in your health and your ability to fully live the life you have earned.

By following the OTM plan, you can keep yourself healthy and fit with lots of energy to do whatever you want and really enjoy your life. You will lose weight, look great, and live a happier, healthier life for the rest of your life.

Note to those who already know me:

For those of you who read *Perfect Body*, I want you to know my beliefs about cleansing, fasting, and overall nutrition haven't changed. *Perfect Body* has a following all over the world. *Perfect Body* has found a home in the Netherlands, England, Scotland, Pakistan, Italy, France, Spain, Mexico, Greece, Africa, Japan, China, and Canada

I wrote *Perfect Body* in 1995 based upon the research I did to cure myself, and the practices I adopted that changed my life for the better. It is an approach to living that has worked for me and for many individuals with the courage to take control of their lives.

My desire in writing *Overcoming the Myths of Aging* is to take the same ideas in *Perfect Body* to a broader audience, and in doing so, contribute to improving the lives of even more people. As I faced the realities of aging, I saw in my family, my friends, in acquaintances, and in society around me a greater need than ever before to promote the benefits of better nutrition and a healthier life style. The purpose of the OTM plan is to start people where they are, not make them wrong or set them up for failure, and help them get healthier. The goal is healthier not perfect.

If you want to be perfect, I happen to have already written a book for that too…

BIBLIOGRAPHY
& Resources

Bibliography

Many years ago, as I began looking for answers that would help me recapture my health; I came upon this text on physiology. It forms the basis for many of the core concepts in the *Perfect Body* and *Overcoming the Myths of Aging*, and is still regarded as a definitive text on physiology. Its 10th edition was released in 2006, and I still see this book as the most accurate and clearly written work on physiology available today.

Vander, Sherman, Lucino. Human Physiology. 10th ed. New York: McGraw-Hill, 2006.

In addition, many other works have help to shape my programs for good nutrition, positive thinking, health and exercise. The following are a few of the most influential and interesting.

Mind and Spirit:

Beckwith, Michael. Inspirations of the Heart.
Los Angeles: Agape Global Ventures, 2004.

Carnigie, Dale. How to Win Friends and Influence People.
New York: Pocket, reissue 1990.

Coelho, Paulo. The Alchemist.
San Francisco: Harper, reprinted 1995.

Dyer, Wayne. The Power of Intention.
Carlsbad: Hay House, 2004.

Frankl, Viktor E. Man's Search for Meaning.
New York: Pocket, revised and updated 1997.

Hill, Napoleon. Think and Grow Rich.
San Diego: Aventine Press, reprinted 2004.

Mitchell, Stephen. Tao to Ching.
New York: Harper Perennial, reprinted 1992.

Peal, Norman Vincent. The Power of Positive Thinking.
New York: Ballantine Books, reissue 1996.

Robbins, Anthony. Awaken the Giant Within.
New York: Free Press, reprinted 2003.

Ruiz, Don Miquel. The Four Agreements.
San Rafael: Amber-Allen Publishing, 1997

The Secret. DVD. TS Productions, 2006.

Diet and health:

Klein, David. Self-Healing Colitis and Crohn's.
Sebastopol: Living Nutrition Publications, 2006.

Schindler, Lydia. Understanding the Immune System.
NIH Publication No. 92-529. U.S. Department of Health and
Human Services, 1991.

Shelton, Herbert. Fasting Can Save Your Life.
Tampa: American Natural Hygiene Society, 1964.

Tilden, John H. Toxemia Explained.
Whitefish: Kessinger Publishing, reprinted 1997.

Eyesight:

Bates, William. The Bates Method for Better Eyesight Without Glasses. New York: Henry Holt and Company, 1981.

Huxley, Aldous. The Art of Seeing.
Seattle: Montana Books, 1978.

Quackenbush, Thomas R. Relearning to See.
Berkeley: North Atlantic Books, 1997.

Eye openers:

Eker, Harv. Secrets of the Millionaire Mind.
New York: Harper Collins, 2005.

Grace, Matthew. A Way Out.
New York: Matthew Grace, 2000.

Robbins, John. Diet for a New America.
Wapole: Stillpoint Publishing, 1987.

Schlosser, Eric. Fast Food Nation.
New York: Harper Perennial, 2002.

Weaver, Don. To Love and Regenerate the Earth: Further Perspectives on The Survival of Civilization.
San Francisco: Don Weaver, 2002.

Exercise:

Hanna, Thomas. Somatics.
Cambridge: DaCapo Press, new edition, 2004.

Wittenberg, Henry. Isometrics Instant Exercise.
New York: Universal Publishing, 1970.

Vella, Mark. Anatomy for Strength and Fitness Training.
New York: McGraw-Hill, 2006.

Books:

Gallo, R. <u>Body Ecology</u>.
San Francisco: Gallo Publications, 1994.

Gallo, R. Perfect <u>Body Beyond the Illusion</u>.
San Francisco: Gallo Publications, 2002

Gallo, R. <u>Perfect Body The Raw Truth</u>.
San Francisco: Promotion Publishing, 1997.

Gallo, R. <u>On Your Way to a Healthy Blood Pressure</u>.
San Francisco: Gallo Publications, 2004.

Tapes and CDs

<u>Perfect Body</u>	available on tape	coming soon on CD
<u>Overcoming the Myths of Aging</u>		coming soon on CD
<u>Self Hypnosis</u>	available on tape	coming soon on CD

Check out my website www.roegallo.com for updated publications and availability.